The Art of SelfLove

The Art of SelfLove

LOVING YOURSELF IS THE KEY TO HAPPINESS

FRANK M. LOBSIGER

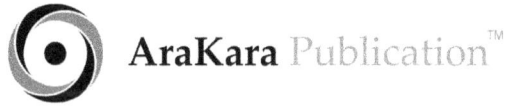

AraKara Publication™

Contact the author at: AraKara Publication, Frank M. Lobsiger, Chemin du Jura 53, 1470 Estavayer-Le-Lac, Switzerland, Phone: ++41 (0) 26 670 3324
E-Mail: FrankLobsiger@TheArtofSelfLove.com

Copyright © 2010 by Frank M. Lobsiger.

ISBN: 978-3-9523605-0-7

Disclaimer Statement
The publisher and author of this book make no medical or psychological claims for its use or effects. This material is not intended to treat, diagnose, advise about, or cure any physical illness or mental disturbance of any kind. If you need medical, psychiatric, or psychological attention or care, please contact your doctor or medical practitioner for professional assistance. The reader is fully responsible for her / his use of the Welcoming-Process™ and the information contained in this book.

*I dedicate this book to
the Source of Love & Happiness,
the Divine,
the One Self,
in & out of which we all live.*

Contents

Introduction

FOR many years I suffered from ongoing self-criticism, self-rejection, and self–abandonment. But most of all I hurt from a lack of *Selflove*.* Having since learned to love myself, I now look back and recognize a remarkable fact: all that pain and hardship was not caused by another person or some ill-fated situation as I had imagined. The greatest pain I have ever known was self-inflicted—generated by the hostile attitude I held towards myself. If self-attack in its many forms also causes pain in your life, then *The Art of Selflove* is written just for you. You see, the negative attitude you hold toward yourself is something you *learned,* and therefore it can be *unlearned* and replaced by a loving and self-affirming attitude.

At the age of seventeen, my habitual self-attacks were so violently hostile and hyper-critical that they eroded almost all of my self-esteem and self-confidence. With a sense of self that was *crushed to pieces,* I found myself truly unhappy. Adding to my misery, feelings of worthlessness alienated me from others and the world. And yet, from the depths of this dark hole, I felt an intense longing to find true happiness, which led me on a journey of self-discovery and self-healing.

Only when I finally decided to love myself, *no matter what,* did my inner war begin to calm down. Step by step I experienced the self-esteem, self-confidence, freedom, and happiness that comes from loving myself; and so will you if you use the key method in this book to cultivate the *Art of Selflove.*

We are so conditioned to look for happiness *out there.* We look to others for love. We chase pleasure, in the form of sex, food, and holidays to make us feel good. We imagine that an attractive partner, a high paying job, a prestigious position, financial security, a luxurious home, and a fancy car will bring

---

*The term "*Selflove*" is written intentionally in one word – without a hyphen – throughout this book to emphasize the innate unity of "Self" and "Love" in its essential state of being. Selflove also stands for the process of cultivating a conscious and loving relationship with oneself. (see glossary, p. 195)

lasting happiness. As you likely know from experience, the initial *kick* that comes with obtaining anything eventually wears off and—*here you are again*—you feel as incomplete and needy as before. Lasting fulfillment eludes you. Regardless of how successful, rich, appreciated, and loved you are, sooner or later you will end up face to face with yourself. You cannot run away from yourself, because the one human being you will always have to live with is *you*. And if fear, frustration, or boredom does not kill your cheerfulness, then some unexpected circumstance—bad luck or a crisis—will take away your *external source of happiness*. What do you do then? How do you deal with loss?

I was faced with this exact challenge a few years ago when my marriage ended and I lost my outer source of happiness—the human being I loved the most at the time. Six months after my wife and I separated, I was still suffering tremendously. I missed her loving presence, her nurturing affection and tenderness; being apart from her was an aching wound that would not heal. Every night, when I came home after work and entered my empty house, I was newly confronted with feelings of loneliness and separation. On one of those nights I found myself wondering, "What do I do now? Do I search for another woman who will give me sweet love and make me forget this pain?" It was clear to me then that seeking comfort in another woman's arms was more an escape than a solution. I knew it was my job to take care of my hurt—even though I felt isolated.

At the lowest point, I began to ask myself, "What is really important in life? What is it that makes life worth living?" The answer came readily: *love*. One question chased the next, "What is love? Is love something that I can voluntarily create or is it something that just comes and goes as it wants?" I was full of questions that I truly could not answer. "Is love and loving the same? If not, what is the difference? How do you love? What do you do when you love? How does one love another? When do you feel loved?" This spontaneous inquiry led me to the fundamental question, *"How do you love yourself?"*

Intuitively I knew that *my own loving* was the prescription for healing my heartache. But I had no clue how to love myself in a practical and tangible way. Up to this point I'd always been more concerned with *being loved* than *loving* because I expected love and the resulting happiness to come from another human being. Of course I did my best to be a loving man with my spouse so that she felt happy in my presence and would continue showering me with her love. In this dynamic of loving her in order to be loved in return, I had never really learned to love myself. On the contrary: my dependency on my partner's love kept increasing, as did my fear of the hurt and dismay that would come should I lose it one day. I had never examined my belief that love comes from the outside, and I had no experience of how to access it on the inside.

We invest tens, hundreds, even thousands of hours learning how to walk, how to speak, how to read, how to calculate, how to ride a bike, how to drive a car, how to play an instrument, how to speak a foreign language, how to use a computer, how to be proficient in your work, and how to master countless other skills. But have you ever spent even one hour learning how to love yourself? Do you know how to relate to yourself in conscious and loving way?

Ask yourself sincerely; can you remember if anybody ever taught you about Selflove? If you are like most people the answer is, "No." We expect that it's a given—you either have it or you don't, like an ear for music—when really Selflove is a skill that can be learned. How can you expect to love yourself if you've never learned what is involved? Sometimes human beings like to believe they know how to do something simply because they are grown-ups. To use an analogy, this would be like assuming that just because you are an adult you know how to play the piano. And then when I ask you to play a song for me, you suddenly realize, "Oh, I don't really know how to play the piano!" The situation is not all that different when it comes to loving yourself.

Isn't it strange that you learn so many things, but never learn how to love yourself and be your own best friend? Well, you are not alone. Most people are completely in the dark when it comes to the practical application of Selflove, especially during tough times when you need your own loving the most.

Fortunately, the love and happiness we all search for is not out there, not in another, but *inside ourselves*. Everyone has an innermost Self, which is the true source of love and happiness. Unfortunately during the course of your life your essential qualities—such as love, joy, peace, creativity, aliveness, humor, enthusiasm, spontaneity, and courage— are obscured by self-hatred that manifests as self-criticism, self-rejection, and self-abandonment. The greater your self-attack, the less you are able to express your essential qualities. As a result you feel cut off from your inner center, your Self, which leaves you feeling profoundly unhappy. Self-attack is like a poison that progressively kills off happiness while spreading its damaging influence. First it destroys your self-esteem and self-worth, then your self-confidence and ability to successfully pursue and achieve your goals. If this harmful cycle continues it can lead you to believe that you are worthless, powerless, and damned to live a miserable and insignificant life. This is not true! This negative, self-destructive behavior can be reversed and transformed into a positive, self-affirming, and self-loving cycle, and this book will show you how.

Probably, like me, you were never given an instruction manual on how to love and relate to yourself in a conscious and loving way. This book is such a manual and is the result of my own *Selflove-journey*. At its heart is the Welcoming-Process—the culmination of more than twenty years of conscious, personal research through introspection and self-analysis. This method draws on knowledge and insights gained in numerous professional trainings in the healing arts, countless books, dozens of courses and workshops, thousands of hours of therapy sessions with clients, and many years of daily yoga practice. The Welcoming-Process is a powerful, practical, and straightforward 3-step method that will show you how to cultivate the Art of Selflove in your own life. This process is a lifetime skill, like writing or reading. Once you get a clear hold of it, it is yours forever.

I believe that the main purpose of life is to grow your ability to love. The ultimate practice then, is to love yourself—*no matter what*. What better place to learn the *art of loving* than inside yourself, in your own bodymind? And before you know it, this love naturally and gradually, step by step, *spills over* from you to others as well. In this moment you will realize that Selflove is the best foundation for *loving another* and creating fulfilling relationships. Therefore the greatest gift you can give yourself, your loved ones, and the world as a whole is to begin to love yourself.

Since the Welcoming-Process has brought greater love and happiness to my friends, my clients, my *Selflove-Training* participants, and me, I know it will do the same for you. May you enjoy your Selflove-journey with the Welcoming-Process and discover for yourself that *loving yourself is the key to happiness!*

How to use this book

THIS book is intended as a practical manual with step-by-step instructions that teach you how to love yourself – how to become your own best friend. In addition, *The Art of Selflove* can be used as a source of inspiration and insight; it can help you better understand yourself, other people, and human nature. Central to this guide is a simple, powerful method called the Welcoming-Process that is introduced in Part Three. Part One and Part Two of the book lay the groundwork with specific terms and concepts that assist you in deepening your understanding of where you are now and where you can go with the Welcoming-Process. For this reason, I recommend that you read the book in a sequential manner, starting with chapter 1. If you cannot wait to find out how the actual method works, I invite you to jump ahead to Part Three, the heart of the book, and familiarize yourself with the three basic steps of the *Selflove-process*. Once you have read Part Three, you would do well to start with chapter 1 and read the book in succession as to comprehend the method-specific terms* and fully absorb the foundational information and diagrams of this book. For clarity and ease of use should you need a quick review of what you've learned, I have placed crucial information and guidelines in textboxes, diagrams, and bold printed statements.

* In the glossary, on p. 193 - you will find a list with explanations of the most important terms.

PART ONE

"Getting to Know Yourself"

CHAPTER 1

An Early Glimpse of Selflove

"The highest power and happiness proceeds from loving all."
Babaji Nagaraj

CARL Gustav Jung, Swiss psychiatrist and originator of Jungian or Analytical Psychology, calls them *big dreams:* those emotionally vibrant, intensely revealing glimpses into the vastness beyond ordinary reality that stay with us throughout our lives. These dreams are transpersonal and archetypal in nature; they communicate shared themes and offer healing for the individual as well as for the collective. I had such a dream when I was six years old.

THE TEMPLE DREAM

I am standing in front of an impressive flight of stairs that leads up to a monumental white temple. Each step appears to be about two feet high. It is clear to me that this is—without question—the most sacred temple in Greece and in the entire antique world. I am determined to climb the stairs and go up to the entrance. As I get closer to the huge portal of the temple, a voice resounds in my mind, "You cannot go up to this temple. You are not allowed to do so, because this holy place was built only for spiritually advanced beings, such as yogis, seers, and saints."

Although I hear the words of this voice very clearly, I remain determined, "I want to go up to the entrance of this temple and nothing is going to stop me!" After having climbed about thirty steps, I stand in front of a two winged wooden entrance door. On each side of the wings I see ornamented white marble pillars that hold up the triangular shaped structure of the roof. The pillars are about ninety feet high.

Standing at the entrance, the same voice begins to speak to me in an even louder and firmer tone, "You have to turn around. Go back! You are not qualified to enter this sacred temple. Only truly holy men are allowed to go in. You have not reached this state of wisdom and sainthood required. Turn around!" Deep inside of me I know the voice speaks the truth, for I am not a wise man and for sure not a saint. This temple was established for holy and wise men, not for a lad like me. Nevertheless, something in me feels driven to continue. A man in white robes walks up the stairs not far from where I'm standing. He moves with such grace and lightness that it seems as if he is levitating up the steps. He comes closer, but before I can see his face a *hush* comes over the scene and he disappears into the temple. I know in my bones that he is an exceptional being, truly a human embodiment of the divine. I come to the door but the handle is too high for me to reach so I push against the right wing of the portal just as the saint did. To my surprise, it opens easily.

I look upward in awe at the row of gigantic stone pillars that stand about two hundred feet apart to the right and left of me. My eyes follow the pillars higher and higher as they reach into the infinite enormity of space. Clearly, this is a temple that no man could have built. Gradually it dawns on me: this temple is a gateway, a passage into another dimension. While the bustling city of Greece enjoys a bright sunny day just outside the temple doors, inside I can see the infinity of outer space spreading out above me in all of its immensity as the night sky.

The ground beneath me is entirely covered with flat stone plates. A soft light that seems to come from nowhere permeates the space around me making it possible to see even though it is dark inside the temple. My intention is set and I follow the hallway deeper into the heart of the temple, passing pillar after pillar. Again I hear the voice: "Turn around! You have to stop! You cannot go on. This is forbidden territory! You have no authorization to be here!" I ignore the voice and keep walking. My sense of time and space are completely lost in the vastness that surrounds me.

Finally, I come to the end of the long hallway of pillars and stand at the entrance of a gigantic plaza. I stop briefly but decide to keep going even though the voice inside me keeps *shouting*, "Stop! Turn around!" I reach the middle of the plaza where I see a round circle—about two and a half feet in diameter—has been chiseled into a stone plate. As I reach the perimeter of the stone circle, I stand still. I have a deep inner knowing, "This stone circle is the heart of the temple, the *holy of holies*. This is the reason why this temple was built in the first place and why the wise and holy men come here." Before I finish gathering my thoughts, the voice resounds again: "Go back! Turn around!" The voice is even more resolute than before as it warns: "Don't dare even think of stepping into the circle. Only those who have reached the highest level of enlightenment and self-realization are allowed to stand in this holy circle, the temple's heart."

I hesitate while I muster all my courage. Then I step into the sacred circle. The voice becomes totally still. I am full of excitement, wondering what will happen next. At once a column of light from high above me fills out the inside of the stone circle. In the most gentle way imaginable, the light begins to penetrate each cell of my body, transfusing every particle and all of my existence—every sensation, every emotion, every thought, everything I have ever experienced, felt or desired throughout time. My entire being completely relaxes and fills with the most exquisite sensation of warmth, sweetness, and ecstasy. "I am home! Finally!" I am absorbed in bliss, bathed in the light of love, and I realize that I am standing in the presence of love itself.

The joy and fulfillment of this instant is beyond description. I am completely at peace and filled with inexpressible gratitude and joy. Love is all that exists. All is perfect in the presence of this divine light. *ALL IS LOVE – ABSOLUTE GOODNESS.*

Then at some point I find myself thinking, "There is *really nothing* that I could still desire anymore." All the riches and pleasures of the universe could not tempt me to step out of the circle of love. I had no wish left, except one: to fully, totally, and forever merge with this divine light. "Yes, this is my final and ultimate desire to be one with You, Beloved Lovelight!"

All of a sudden, I look at my body and realize there are spots of darkness, *shadow patches,* that won't let the light go through. In this very moment the blatant truth of my situation becomes fully apparent to me. Intuitively I understand the implication of the darkness in my body. It is the toughest truth I ever had to look straight in the face. The dark shadow-patches are the parts of myself that I have judged, rejected, and not yet learned to love. Anything that I ever hated and despised in myself or someone else, I can now see in the form of dark spots in my translucent body. It is clear to me that I cannot become one with love until I welcome, love, and heal these shadow patches, so that they can transform back into light. Only then will I be able to fully merge with the Divine Lovelight forever.

Then it dawns on me, "Oh, this is why the voice in me kept insisting I turn around!" It did not want to hold me back. It wanted to protect me from this excruciating pain of being unable to unite with the lovelight completely. I knew I had no option but to make the most painful decision ever: to step out of the stone circle and keep on walking straight ahead, across the plaza, down the hallway of stone pillars, and out the door on the other side of the temple.

I wake up, deeply moved and profoundly aware that I must learn to love myself. I realize that every aspect of myself that I have ever rejected, repressed, hated, feared, or judged wants and needs to be loved. Only if I learn to love all my shadow patches can they transform back into light and only then will I be able to merge with the lovelight.

Since I had this dream at such a young age, I did not know how I would fulfill this great task and learn to love myself. Now decades later, I have the privilege to offer you the Welcoming-Process, a simple and practical method for cultivating the Art of Selflove.

I created this process in order to overcome my own relentless self-attack, as well as my dependency on another person's love; my own suffering forced me to come up with a solution. When you apply this powerful, elegant, and straightforward *technique* in your life, you will begin to love yourself ever more fully. As you transform your shadow patches step by step, you will find that this process *frees your inner light*, which is the true source of love and happiness within you.

"There is no weapon more powerful for the realization of truth than the one of accepting yourself."
Swami Prajnanpad

CHAPTER 2

Love & Happiness

**"Love is the central flame of the universe, nay the very fire itself.
The essence of love, while elusive, pervades everything, fires the
heart, stimulates the emotions, renews the soul and proclaims
the Spirit. Only love knows love, and love only knows love."**
Ernest Holmes

YOU, me, everybody yearns for love. Why? Because whenever you feel love you feel truly happy and whole. In this moment all your desires, all your wishes are fulfilled. In the presence of love your worries and your sorrows begin to dissolve. You feel totally at peace as though you have come *home*. You are one with your very Self, the Divine in you, the core of your being. One with love you are overflowing with bliss and ultimate happiness. In other words, love and happiness go hand in hand.

Love is the source of happiness.

Love is always a subjective experience, unique to the man or woman who feels it. Deep inside you know the nature of love. Love is an inner experience, not something objective that can be quantified or looked at from the outside. If you want to know the flavor and texture of vanilla ice cream, you have to taste it.

The best things in life cannot be explained; they can only be experienced. The same is true of happiness. No one can tell you what happiness is because it cannot be described. Can you describe light to someone that has been sitting in a dark room all his life?

"If you could feel even a particle of Divine Love, so great would be your joy, so overpowering – you could not contain it."
Paramahansa Yogananda

AN INVITATION TO REMEMBER— THE HAPPIEST MOMENT OF YOUR LIFE

I invite you to take a moment, go inside, and consider the following question:

"What is the happiest moment/experience you can remember?"

I have posed this question in the present tense intentionally because I want you to re-live the moment anew, as if you are experiencing it for the very first time. Once you bring the moment fully to mind, allow the questions below to further awaken your memory. Take as much time as you like. Plunge deeply into this moment of grace. As you dive deep into this memory, you give yourself the gift of connecting with your inner happiness.

- Where are you?
- What is the environment like?
- How is the atmosphere?
- What are you doing?
- What are you feeling?
- What do you sense in your body?
- How do you feel right now as this memory unfolds and takes shape in your inner world?
- How would you describe the overall experience as you remember and reconnect with the happiest moment of your life?

THE ETERNAL SEARCH FOR LOVE & HAPPINESS

**"Happiness is the meaning and the purpose of life,
the whole aim and end of human existence."**
Aristotle

The search for love and happiness is the driving force in everybody's life. You look for happiness in relationships, money, possessions, status, achievement, and any number of experiences that promise satisfaction. Some endeavors attract you more than others because they seem to hold more potential for future happiness. Unfortunately we often end up frustrated and disillusioned in our pursuit because we confuse pleasure with happiness.

Let's take this inquiry a step further. Where do you look for love and happiness in your life? The way you like to spend your free time is a good pointer. Most of us expect the greatest love and happiness to come from a love relationship. You feel a deep instinctual urge to find and merge with *the one*. Hollywood movies, TV commercials, romantic novels, all tell you that you need to find that one because he or she will make you happy for the rest of your life. Reality seems to contradict this romantic notion, however, and far more relationships lead to heartbreak and disappointment than to happily ever after.

What do you do when your partnership/marriage turns sour or comes to an end? Do you go out and look for a new partner—a better, more perfect one—who will not fail you and make you unhappy a second time? If you are less optimistic or somewhat disheartened about finding "the one", then you will be content if the *new one* does not have the same flaws your previous partner had—too much of this, too little of that, you name it.

You may decide to stop the search and resign from romantic involvements altogether. People who give up the search for love and happiness often become disheartened and depressed. If you are reading this book, it's likely that you haven't given up; otherwise you would not bother reading these words. You are still searching and you keep looking for the best. You may even find that you are quite happy without a romantic partner, and yet in your heart you still feel a certain longing. This is your nature: you cannot really give up the search until you have found a reliable source of love. But where do you look for it?

A TRAGIC SEARCH — YOU LOOK FOR LOVE/HAPPINESS WHERE IT IS NOT

**"If God/Goddess wanted to play hide and seek with man/
woman, then God/Goddess would hide inside of man/woman,
because this is the last place a human being will ever search."**
Asian Saying

The tragic part of this whole search is that you keep looking for love where it is not and where it will never be—*out there.* Happiness does not come from out there. It comes from within, from the center of your being. What you are really looking for is your innermost Self, capitalized. This Self is the very source of love and happiness.

Have you ever found lasting happiness out there? Could you hold on to it? Do you know anyone who has? Most likely you do not. It is a human tendency to associate love and happiness with someone or something in the outer world. Trying to possess and hold on to happiness in the form of a lover or some favorite object is like trying to grasp water with your hands. It is a futile endeavor because eventually it will run through your fingers and be gone. Likewise it is the same with happiness. The outer world cannot give it to you; it can, at best, support you in experiencing the love and happiness that already exists within.

Everything that assists you in establishing or deepening the connection with your true Self will increase the amount of love and happiness available to you. Loving people, precious belongings, favorable circumstances, and pleasurable activities can support you in getting in touch with your inner Self, and yet they are not the source of your happiness.

Some people who seem to have everything in their lives—a good job, a loving, attractive partner, a healthy body, a comfortable home, a supportive family, loyal friends—still feel unhappy, maybe even miserable. How is this possible? Because they feel cut off from the Self, which is the seat of love and happiness. Nobody and nothing out there can ever make you feel happy or loved when you feel disconnected from your very Self. Every time you feel unhappy or miserable it is because you have lost touch with your innermost center.

In the foreword to *The Philosophy of Love* by Haridas Chaudhuri: "Who is abandoning us? Certainly not Love. We must stop blocking this most fundamental universal energy from coming into our lives by obsessively looking for it in every other direction but the right one. We misplace our priorities in seeking a true experience of love when we blindly search for it horizontally, from others, rather than letting it flow into us from the very core of life itself."*5

"Do oysters know the value of their pearls,
Or space the reach of its infinity?
As the Moon knows nothing of the moonlight,
Men do not know their own divinity."
Excerpt from the Tablets of Shambala

"We are not human beings having a spiritual experience.
We are spiritual beings having a human experience."
Theilhard de Chardin

So, rather than continuing to chase after love and happiness out there, let's begin to look inside your very Self.

YOUR INNER SUN -
THE SOURCE OF LOVE & HAPPINESS

"He who sparkles in your eyes, who lights the heavens and hides
in the souls of all creatures is God, your Self."
Siva Yogaswami of the Natha Sampradaya

"Love is the Self. The Self doesn't love. The Self is Love."
Lester Levenson

The source of love and happiness lives within you as your very Self. It is the *Divine Self* in and out of which you, me, everyone, and everything live. Your Self is the heart of your being at the very core of who you truly are. I call this Divine Self in you the *Inner Sun*. Your Inner Sun is true source of all love and happiness. The Inner Sun is the center of your life and your very existence.

All essential qualities such as love, happiness, peace, harmony, vitality, health, beauty, intelligence, wisdom, humor, creativity… and all others emerge from your Inner Sun. The essential qualities are like rays emerging and radiating out from your Inner Sun. Each ray of your Inner Sun warms and lights up everything that it touches with its unique quality.

To use an analogy, your Inner Sun is like the colorless, white light that contains and unifies all spectral colors within its nature. When the white light passes through a prism it disperses into spectral light, and the various rainbow colors appear. In our example each spectral or rainbow color represents one unique essential quality, whereas the Inner Sun stands for the white light.

> **"Love emerges from you because it is in you."**
> Daniel Odier

> **"Throughout the ages, various spiritual teachings have affirmed unconditional and unlimited love to be at the very core of the universe and that from which all life radiates."**
> Dionne Marx

The ancient sages and yogis from India have a special word to describe the Self: *Sat-cit-ananda*. Translated into English, *sat* means existence, *cit* means consciousness, and *ananda* means bliss.*12 Sat-cit-ananda is the expression of what the yogis realize in deepest meditation when they enter the state of union with their innermost Self. Satcitananda is what you really are—a *Sun of Existence-Consciousness-Bliss*.

The Inner Sun is eternal and indestructible. This truth is beautifully expressed in the Bhagavad-Gita when the warrior Arjuna is instructed by Lord Krishna to prepare himself for battle. Here is the passage in which Krishna teaches Arjuna about the Self, which he calls *He-the Dweller*: "As a man casting off worn-out garments, takes other new ones, so the dweller in the body casting off worn-out bodies, takes others that are new. He is uncleavable; he cannot be burned, he cannot be wetted, nor can he be dried. He is eternal, all-pervading, stable, immovable, ever the same."*13

C.G. Jung writes about the Self: "The self is not only the centre but also the whole circumference which embraces both consciousness and unconscious;

it is the center of this totality…"*14 - "The self is our life's goal, for it is the completest expression of that fateful combination we call individuality."*15

"…the source of happiness in life, that is, the ever existent inner joy of the soul."
Marshall Govindan & Jan Ahlund

I invite you to take this step from the divine sphere of love to the level of human experience with me. In the following chapter I will show you what it is that prevents you from experiencing love and happiness. I will further give you a human model, a sort of inner roadmap, that will enhance your understanding of *exactly what it is* that blocks you from experiencing your Inner Sun.

CHAPTER 3

The Source of Unhappiness - Your Inner War

**"Men are at war with each other because
each man is at war with himself."**
Francis Meehan

THE greatest pain and suffering in your life is caused by the ongoing *inner war* you wage against yourself. This recurring, enduring battle can even be constant at times, and not only is it immensely hurtful, it also blocks the rays of your Inner Sun, the love and happiness at your core. But the inner war need not be unending, for it is entirely self-perpetuated as you will see in this chapter. To help you understand the causes and conditions that feed the war within you, I will present a simple human model called the *3-layered self.* This will help you get to know yourself better and gain perspective on what happens with all the unwanted aspects of yourself that you criticize, reject, and repress. You will understand how the *shadow layer,* also called your *shadow self,* is created and how it cuts you off from your Divine Self. Furthermore, you will read about the *happiness killer,* the *inner critic,* and the *ideal self.*

THE 3-LAYERED SELF

The diagram below represents three fundamental aspects or layers of a human being. The outermost layer is the called the *mask,* or *social self;* it is the conscious part of your personality. The secondary or middle layer is the *shadow self* and is the unconscious part of your persona. The primary, innermost layer represents your Inner Sun—the Divine Self with all its essential qualities.

This model draws on the work of Wilhelm Reich (1897 -1953), the

Austrian psychiatrist and psychoanalyst who is widely regarded as the father of modern body-oriented psychotherapy. I have modified and synthesized what Reich conceptualized as the *3 existential layers*2 within the human being according to my understanding of human nature and insights gained from working in private practice since 1996.

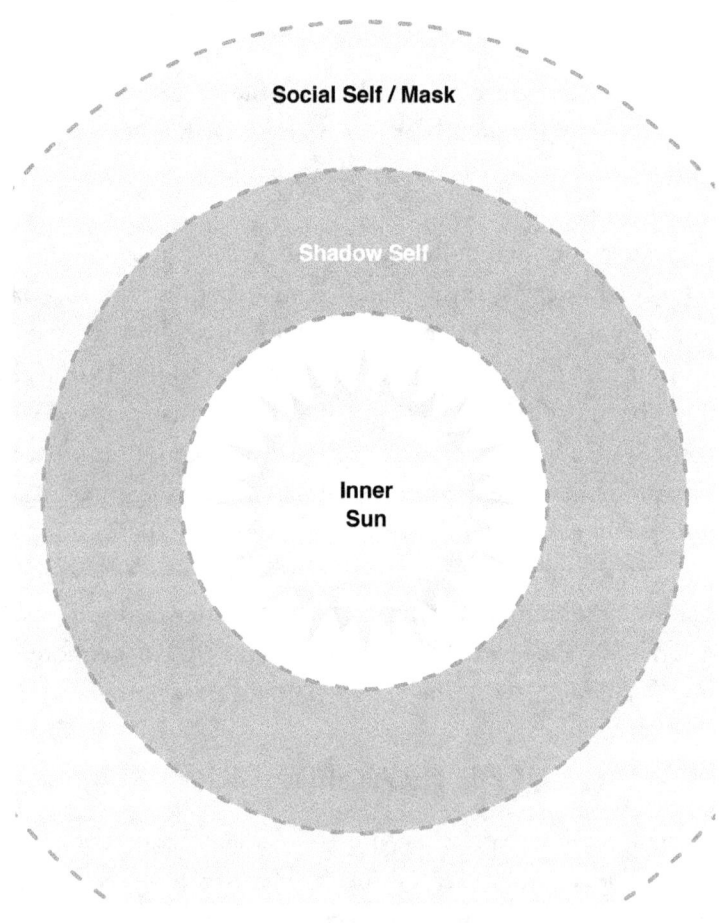

Diagram of the 3-layered self

It is important to mention that no model or a diagram can ever fully capture your personal experience. At best, this model can be used as a roadmap to show you where you are and where you are going. The intention of the model of the 3-layered self is to assist you in understanding yourself better by mapping your inner and outer world. Each layer is *alive*, and has a degree of fluidity to it. As you evolve, they change and shift as well.

To be loved or not to be loved — a question of life or death

As a baby, you are born fully open and undefended, with a thin and sensitive skin that is in need of a loving touch and a helplessly dependent physical body that requires protection and care. You instinctively know that your survival depends on your parents' ability to nurture you and tend to your needs. You are completely vulnerable and reliant on your providers—*whether they recognize how vulnerable you are or not.* Then, one day, you feel inwardly distressed and you scream and kick against your mother, which makes her very upset. She looks at you with an angry face, scolds you in a loud voice, puts you in your crib with a brisk motion, and leaves you all alone in the room. You cannot understand this sudden separation and begin crying desperately. But Mommy does not come back. You feel entirely abandoned and terrified.

It is natural for a child to blame her or himself for parental rejection or punishment and to conclude *on a feeling level:* "I did something bad," or— even worse—to begin to believe that he has some kind of innate badness. Such an *emotional conclusion* might be: "Mommy is not coming back because I did something bad. She does not love me anymore because I am so bad. And now she is punishing me by staying away from me. I will die without her loving care!"

The pain of being rejected or ignored, of not being loved by his parents seems unbearable to the child and is truly horrifying. He is convinced that if he were to fully allow himself to feel this pain, it would destroy him. To be loved or not to be loved means to be or not to be—to live or to die. It is a question of life or death. As a result you decide that you will do whatever it takes to be loved by your mother since this is essential for you to survive. You make a solemn promise to yourself: "From now on I am only going to be good. I will hold back what is bad and no longer express it or let her see it. I will do what

Mommy likes so that she loves me again and keeps taking care of me." This decision leads to the birth of your mask.

THE MASK

Each family, society, and culture has a unique set of rules, guidelines, or social codes that determine appropriate behavior. The mask is the most superficial part of your social self and your conscious personality. It incorporates all these social rules and interacts with the outside world. It is called the mask, or the *false self*, because it expresses only the socially acceptable side of you and conceals the rest of your personality.

Your mask knows exactly how you *should be* and how you have to behave in order to be accepted by your family, friends, co-workers, or whomever you are interacting with. It helps you to fit in, to behave like a normal, well-adapted human being, and to be a good citizen. Your social self also prevents you from *acting out* your negative, socially offensive thoughts and feelings. For example, your mask may hide a miserable mood or prevent you from expressing anger toward others. The mask makes sure that you control yourself and treat others in a civilized and respectful way, even if you don't feel like doing so. The formation of the mask allows you to develop these necessary social skills.

Growing up, you were trained how to behave by your parents, family members, friends, neighbors, teachers, and schoolmates. In other words, the important people in your social environment showed you how you *should be*. They taught you how you should act, what kind of demeanor and personal expressions are acceptable or desirable, and which ones are not. At some point you realized that you were only lovable if you behaved in a way that your parents liked and approved of. The *good child* in you that displayed the right behavior was loved and got rewarded, whereas the *bad child* that did the wrong thing was criticized and punished. In this manner, you were conditioned by your parents and your social surroundings to be a good child. "Please them," became your mandate, albeit an unconscious one.

The mask is most of all a *defense mechanism* that serves a protective function for your social self. The basic intention of the mask is to keep you *safe*. It protects you from both internal and external threats. Externally, the mask serves to protect you from hurtful criticism, rejection, and punishment by allowing you to hide from the outer world all that you consider bad, including your sensitivity, vulnerability, neediness, dependency, insecurity, anxiety, as well as any *reactive aspects* that might attack, blame, act out, run away, or withdraw when they feel threatened. Instead of showing what you really feel inside, you put on a false overlay to conceal what you now deem "undesirable" aspects of your personality. Internally, the mask keeps you safe by covering up all your internal conflicts, your pain and suffering. Your personality believes that all the early childhood hurts have the power to destroy you. Therefore all memories of having been attacked, rejected, and abandoned, including all of your shortcomings and anxieties, have to be repressed and forgotten about. It is the goal of the mask to guarantee your survival, by fending off all experiences in the inner and outer world that trigger fear or distress. Anything that threatens to annihilate you, especially if you were to experience it in its full intensity, needs to be avoided.

But what happens to all the hidden, rejected, and unloved aspects within you? Where do they go?

REPRESSION

**The more you have repressed,
the more likely you are to feel depressed.**

Every experience and every facet of your personality that you repress goes *underground* and lives on in *secrecy*, hidden away from your conscious awareness. Nothing that you deny or disown will ever disappear. Your mask suppresses all the *bad* experiences and aspects within you that threaten your sense of safety. Repressed, they continue their concealed existence in the *cellar of your subconsciousness*.

Getting rid of unwanted experiences by repressing them is a common human practice. This strategy of repression is rooted in the belief that suppressing what feels uncomfortable, stressful, or frightening will make it magically disappear from your inner or outer world. Unfortunately, this is nothing but wishful thinking. As you know from your own life experience: there is nothing you can run away from or suppress forever. Because what you escape from remains within you and what you repress is always a part of you.

Repression is an ongoing fight that—for some of us—is unrelenting, and this inner battle uses up a tremendous amount of energy. A huge portion of your life force is consumed when you continuously have to push down the rejected aspects of your personality so that they do not come up to the surface of your conscious mind. It is a natural law that what you fight, fights back; what you push down, pushes back up. To use a simple analogy, let's imagine that each time you repress a discarded aspect of yourself you push down a ping-pong ball under water. Keeping one ping-pong ball under water uses up a little bit of your energy. Over the course of your life, you need ever more energy just to keep all the accumulated ping-pong balls under water, below the surface of your awareness. Every year you have less energy available to pursue your goals, to be yourself, to enjoy life and the company of others, because the inner pressure and conflict from repressing your shadow self becomes ever more intense. Your mask needs to hijack more and more of your vital energy to keep these ping-pong balls from popping up to the surface and revealing their content.

> **"We can better practice self-acceptance when we understand that it is not unwanted feelings that impair healthy functioning but the denial and disowning of those feelings."**
> Nathaniel Branden

THE SHADOW SELF — YOUR IMPRISONED SELF

The shadow self is a common term that I use in this context to highlight all the aspects and experiences of yourself that you reject, deny, and repress. Susan Thesenga, author of *The Undefended Self*, calls this part of the psyche the *lower self*. She writes: "Beneath the mask is the lower self, or source of negativity, destructiveness, separateness within us, which is the true cause of our unhappiness. The lower self is usually unconscious, in whole or in part, because it is hard to admit we have a destructive, negative side to our nature. As children we were made to feel ashamed of the lower self, and we feared, that being honest about our negative feelings would cause us to be rejected by our parents. So we covered it over with a mask that we hoped would ensure our lovability."*4

Since the shadow self is largely unconscious, the first step is to become aware of its existence. Do not be dismayed if you know very little about its content at this point. Once you learn the Welcoming-Process, the shadow self will naturally and organically reveal what it contains.

What you reject becomes distorted & ugly

"Even tendencies that might in some circumstances be able to exert a beneficial influence are transformed into demons when they are repressed."
C.G. Jung

Every experience and every aspect that you repress begins to take on an unconscious *shadow existence*. Together all these *shadow parts* form your shadow self, the rejected, unconscious part of your personality. In phases of introspection, while dreaming or meditating you bring awareness to it and this, in turn, enables you to get an impression of its contents. But hidden away—unknown to the light of your conscious awareness—this rejected self of yours and all its repressed experiences lives an isolated existence.

Carl Gustav Jung who coined the term *the shadow*, defines it as follows: "The shadow personifies everything that the subject refuses to acknowledge about himself and yet is always thrusting itself upon him directly or indirectly – for instance, inferior traits of character and other incompatible tendencies."*6 In another paragraph he says: "The shadow is that hidden, repressed, for the most part inferior and guilt-laden personality..."*7

Life's intention is to flow. In the flow of life there is renewal, health, and harmony. If you are in the flow your life force, your vitality that emerges from the Inner Sun flows freely through your bodymind[1]. The freer the inner flow the happier and more whole you feel.

Your instinctual impulses, needs, desires, emotions, movements, and sounds, including all other forms of expression that are met with non-attendance or rejection, accumulate inside your bodymind and begin to build a *shadow layer*[2]. What is suppressed begins to degenerate and become deformed; in time these isolated parts may grow ugly, negative, even destructive.

Occasionally you might wake up from a nightmare where a monster

---

[1] The term bodymind expresses the unity of the interplay between the physical body and the mind/psyche, as well as the interdependence between the physiological and psychological processes.

[2] In Reich's model the shadow layer is called the secondary layer. Eva Pierrakos, the originator of the Pathwork, calls it the lower self.

or some demon-like creature is chasing you and wants to kill you. This is the result of repression; it is what happens when an instinct, a vital need, an intense emotion, or an intuitive message is being repressed by your conscious mind. Imagine you were locked up in a dark dungeon for weeks, months, years, or even decades. Although you once were a normal human being, you will become filthy and deformed, an ugly looking freak that behaves in strange ways.

Received with hostility and locked up inside, what was originally positive, natural and healthy becomes negative, perverted and destructive. Aliveness turns into fear, lust into shame, need into frustration, aggression into rage, sadness into despair, anxiety into panic, hurt into numbness, passion into craziness, longing into depression, needing into demanding, wanting into violence, intense sensation into overwhelmed paralysis, and so on. These originally innocent, instinctual and vitality-affirming manifestations have become twisted and deformed through repression. These dark ominous patches make up your shadow self. The totality of your inner negativity is ultimately a consequence of your defense against the fear of pain and annihilation. Unlike a normal prisoner, your suppressed life force cannot die; it survives—buried alive in the subconscious of your bodymind.

> **"If we suppress emotion, there is still a negative trace.
> Suppression is a manifestation of aversion. It occurs through
> tightening something inside of ourselves, putting something
> behind a door and locking it, forcing part of our experience into
> the dark where it waits, seemingly hostile, until the appropriate
> secondary cause calls it out."**
> Tenzin Wangyal Rinpoche

Your Inner Sun

The Inner Sun Always Shines.

As mentioned in the second chapter, the core of your being is your Inner Sun, the source of love and happiness. The Inner Sun represents your Divine Self, the seat of your life force, your vitality, your talents, your gifts, all your essential qualities, such as harmony, intelligence, creativity, compassion, joy, beauty, patience, and playfulness to name a few. Every time a ray of your Inner Sun shines forth, your bodymind is permeated by its essential quality. Symbolically speaking the green ray may infuse you with the essential quality of peacefulness, the red ray with courage or passion. Potentially you contain all essential qualities, yet some are more easily accessible to you than others. You can easily see this in children. One child is naturally more physical, outgoing, active, adventurous, courageous, and fiery. Another child is more introverted, intellectual, imaginative, artistic, and reflective. Each of us is born with a dominant set of essential qualities. Your essential qualities are uniquely yours and identify you as you just as clearly as the shape of your face, the colors of your eyes, or the lines on your fingertips. Often you don't even recognize your own essential qualities for when they flow through you, it is effortless, natural and easy. You feel free, happy and light. You are in the flow.

Other people might have similar essential qualities, yet nobody will have the exact same mixture as you. This is why each of us is irreplaceable and one of a kind. What others love in you and what you love in others are the essential qualities embodied and expressed by that person. When you say, "I love her beautiful face" then you love the way the essential quality of beauty expresses itself in that person's face. When you like how someone fights for a just cause, then you are touched by that person's essential quality of courage, uprightness, truthfulness, or integrity. The description you use is unimportant; what counts is the conscious recognition of the essential quality, the unique ray that emerges from the Inner Sun.

Do you know what your Essential Qualities are? Well, there is a very easy way to find out.

INVITATION TO RECOGNIZE YOUR ESSENTIAL QUALITIES

I often ask my clients: "How do you know the color of your eyes?" First they wonder, "What a strange question." And then after some reflection they say, "By looking into a mirror." or "Because somebody told me." Yes, that's right you need a *mirror*, either an actual physical mirror or one in the form of another human being. You will never know the colors of your eyes or the look of your face without something or someone mirroring it to you.

Since nobody knows you better than the people who love you and live with you, ask your partner, your best friends, or the members of your family what they love the most in you. Ask what touches them the most about you and what they would miss the most if you were no longer part of their lives. Their answers will help you recognize your essential qualities.

If you decide to ask your friends and family members, make sure to do it in a quiet, relaxed and peaceful moment when you both feel at ease. Take plenty of time for this exchange. From my own experience I know that this sharing, especially if you alternate the roles, can be deeply moving and life transforming. You will learn something about yourself that you were not aware of. Treasure this experience!

YOUR SHADOW SELF SEPARATES YOU FROM YOUR INNER SUN

**"The sun may be covered for the time being with a patch
of cloud, but regardless of its size or thickness, it can never
diminish the sun's resplendence. Gold may remain buried under
the earth for thousands of years, but that cannot destroy its
natural brilliance. It has only to be dug out, for the golden color
to reveal itself."**
Babaji Nagaraj

If you look at the diagram of the 3-layered self on page 32 you can see that the shadow self separates you from your Inner Sun. The shadow layer cuts you off from your innermost Divine Self, the source of love and happiness. It also inhibits the natural *flow* of spontaneous self-expression and health sustaining *self-regulation*[3] of your bodymind. This is the price you pay for repressing all

---

[3] * Self-regulation, see glossary page 195

of the unwanted aspects and experiences in yourself. The mask's repression of your so-called *negativity* gives your conscious personality a superficial sense of safety, and yet you feel split, cut off from *home* and the root of your existence. The real safety you long for comes from feeling connected with your Inner Sun.

The harder the mask works, the thicker the shadow layer grows between your personality and your Inner Sun. This is the painful dilemma that the mask's defense mechanism creates in you. Your shadow self keeps growing in magnitude and blocking the warming rays of your Inner Sun. It is like the atmosphere in a city that gets so polluted with dust particles you can no longer see the sun behind the dark layered sky. This smog layer is like a thick, dark band of haze that forms your inner horizon. The good news is the sun is not affected by the dark sky, but the bad news is you are, because the sun represents your life force. The Inner Sun is who you truly are, but you have lost your ability to consciously access it. As a baby it was so easy and natural for you to unite with this blissful inner center in the arms of your mother after she fed you and took care of all your needs.

Occasionally, without any announcement, there is an opening, a window in the dark sky of your shadow self and the rays of the Inner Sun penetrate your conscious awareness. In these moments of grace, you feel completely happy, filled with love and gratitude for no apparent reason. You cannot explain why or how this is happening to you. It is a gift of life and you feel like the happiest human being on this planet. You feel full, whole, and bathed in the light of your Inner Sun from deep within.

The shadow self is what I encountered in the *Temple Dream* as shadow patches. In the dream, these shadow patches prevented me from merging with the *lovelight*, which is essentially the Inner Sun.

Now, let's explore what hurts you the most and lies at the root of your unhappiness.

The inner critic

"In order to protect ourselves from the pain and the shame of always being found less than we should be, a voice develops within us that echoes the concerns of our parents, our church, or other people who were important to us in our early years. We literally develop a "self", a separate subpersonality, that criticizes us before our parents—or anyone else, for that matter—can!"
Hal & Sidra Stone

"You are stupid. You will never succeed at anything. You deserve no better. You are selfish. You look so ugly. You are too fat. You should be ashamed of yourself. Nobody will ever love you. You have no talent. This is not for you. Who do you think you are? You are such a coward. You are incapable. You are lazy. You should have studied harder, now it's too late. You are too old. Nobody wants you anymore. Why do you even try, you will fail anyway. Someone else can do that much better than you. You are a born failure."

Do some of these statements sound familiar to you? This is the voice of the inner critic.

How do you recognize the inner critic?

The easiest way to recognize the inner critic is to observe the voice in your head that criticizes and judges you. The voice of the inner critic makes you wrong, puts you down, shames and condemns you, as in the statements above. It likes to make absolute proclamations such as, "You will *never* succeed. You will *always* be broke." Any *negative self-talk* that undermines your sense of self-confidence and self-worth is an expression of your inner critic.

This critical and judgmental voice can become so habitual in the background of your head that you are often not aware that it is speaking to you. Whenever you find yourself feeling depressed, discouraged, and miserable you can be sure that the inner critic is showering you with its censoring, judgmental self-talk.

"Of all the judgments that we pass in life, none is as important as the one we pass on ourselves, for that judgment touches the very center of our existence."
Nathaniel Brandon

Becoming a "superman" or "superwoman"

Since your personality is convinced that happiness lies out there—in other people, objects, and possessions—it keeps searching for ever more effective strategies to get what you most crave from the outer world. For this reason your personality creates the inner critic. The inner critic is a potent alley of your mask, faithfully completing and backing up its work. The purpose of the inner critic is to turn you into a *superwoman* or a *superman* by reinforcing your *idealized self.* This intention stems from the basic assumption that if you could only become an ideal version of yourself, everyone (including you) would be happy. The mask is convinced that an ideal you would be able to command all the security, love, and satisfaction you want.

The ideal self

The inner critic's intention is to push you into becoming an *ideal self*—the best version of you possible—in order to impress or attract the people who are important to you. Depending on the fascination and preferences of your personality, you craft an ideal self that is oriented to either love or power. If you are interested in gaining status and power, you imagine your ideal self to be superior, influential, dominant, ultra-competent, aloof, and full of success appeal. With your ideal self you intend to evoke admiration and awe so that you can take from life what you want. Any form of weakness, insecurity, emotionality, or dependency would contradict or undermine this powerful image. Such impulses must therefore be banished.

On the other hand, if your personality is more interested in *being loved*, you will craft an ideal self along different lines. You might choose the strategy of being sweet, gentle, understanding, insightful, loving, compassionate, patient, helpful, considerate, flexible, mellow, easy-going, or any combination thereof. Your ideal self will do whatever it takes to evoke a loving attitude towards you.

The strategy of your ideal self is to induce a warm and loving response in the other. At the same time, any conduct that creates displeasure, fear, or rejection in the other will be avoided because these would undermine the intention of gaining love.

Of course, any number of variations on these two basic themes can be identified when you look at any group of people. The love-hungry types might have an idealized self that is nuanced toward sexy or spunky or even nerd-like and freaky. The power-hungry types can spin the ideal self with a touch of class, or a touch of brawn, or a stiff dose of tough-guy, or an air of *femme fatale*. Innumerable varieties of *ideal self-versions* exist, and sometimes more than one within a single person.

NOTHING IS EVER GOOD ENOUGH

**"As I peeled away the layers of my life, I realized that
all my craziness, all my pain and difficulties stemmed
from me not valuing myself."**
Oprah Winfrey

The mask uses the inner critic to clear the decks for the ideal self—at least that is its aim, however unattainable. The ideal self is the standard against which every behavior is measured. When your behavior doesn't measure up, the inner critic lets you have it. Any behavior, any character trait, any expression or feeling that is not in keeping with the ideal self image will be penalized. It is the job of the inner critic to uphold the law of the ideal self, and it will criticize, judge, punish—even destroy—as a matter of course.

Your inner critic is geared towards perfection; it wants to turn you into Miss Perfect, or Mr. Wonderful. It may even dream of being a superstar if you live in a celebrity culture. Under this pressure, it will never be satisfied or content with your performance. If you complete something, you could have done it even better. If you do it better, you are still not doing it perfectly. Something always needs to be improved and perfected and thus you are continually criticized and judged. Bottom line: to the inner critic you are never good enough.

INVITATION TO GET TO KNOW YOUR INNER CRITIC & YOUR IDEAL SELF

I invite you to take a moment to consciously reflect on your own inner critic & ideal self.

Remember a situation in your life when you felt your self-confidence was in the process of disappearing and your self-esteem was dropping below zero. Do you remember what happened shortly before you felt this way?

1. What was the content of the self-talk that was going on in your mind?
2. What did the inner critic say to you? Which statement was the most hurtful for you?
3. What kind of ideal self does your inner critic want you to live up to?
4. What are the exact criteria of this ideal self? How should you be and what do you need to avoid at all cost? What is unacceptable and thus needs to be attacked, criticized, and judged in you?

THE INNER CRITIC'S GOOD INTENTION

It is important to recognize the fundamental good intention of the inner critic. By design, it is only trying to keep you *safe* and ensure that you will get the love, control, and satisfaction that you long for. Remember that your inner child created the mask in order to shield itself from the unbearable pain of rejection and abandonment. Behind the inner critic—your mask's protective super weapon—is your terrified inner child that still longs for safety and loving care. The inner critic and the ideal self are simply a composite of all the authoritarian voices you have collected and internalized throughout your life. Each time you don't live up to your ideal self-image, your inner critic freaks out and launches a pitiless self-attack in the form of self-criticism, self-judgment, and self-punishment.

A GOAL YOU CAN NEVER REACH

As an adult you begin to believe who you are is your mask, and that one day—if you work *hard enough*—you will finally become your ideal self. The sober reality, however, is this: *you will never be able to become this ideal self.* It is a false, imaginary construct of your personality that bears little resemblance to your true Self. You pursue a self-image that you would like to be, but have no hope of ever achieving because it is not real. In actual fact you are chasing a mirage, like the optical illusion of water in the desert—a *Fata Morgana*.

The only way you can keep up the illusion of your ideal self-image is by attacking, denying, and repressing anything you say, think, or do that doesn't measure up. This is the source of your ongoing inner war. It is waged against everything in you that is not aligned with the inner critic's idea of your ideal self. As I mentioned before, these attacked, criticized, rejected, and eventually repressed parts live on inside your bodymind, in the shadow layer where they block the rays of your Inner Sun. Unable to feel the core warmth that is essential to who you are, you experience an inner sense of homelessness. With each self-attack of the inner critic the shadow layer blocks the rays of your Inner Sun, the source of love and happiness.

Feeling separate from your Inner Sun triggers anxiety and an inner sense of isolation. The more disconnected you feel from your true Self the more dependent you become on the external world—on possessions, objects, money, status, and people—for your sense of safety and satisfaction. You look outside of you for consolation and comfort in hopes of easing the suffering that comes from feeling cut off from your essential qualities. Insecure and fear-driven, you progressively substitute worry for faith, control for trust, appropriateness for aliveness, performance for spontaneity, adaptation for openness, consumption for creativity, and dominance or submission for loving.

This is the human tragedy: the mask and the ideal self—backed up by the inner critic that should have saved you from pain and suffering, especially as a child—have now become the very cause of your unhappiness. The whole idea of being *safe* and avoiding pain and suffering by becoming your ideal self is a grand misconception. Your inner critic leads an inner battle, a *holy war,* in the name of your ideal self. But it can never win, nor become this unrealistic version of you. In the long run, this tragic illusion causes nothing but suffering in your life.

It is human to feel pain

From childhood on, we try to avoid pain, to cut it out of our lives, although pain and suffering are formative elements in our human growth. Of course it is wise to avoid unnecessary pain and protect yourself against possible accidents or impeding danger, but no one can completely escape from pain or suffering. In the process of living you get hurt. Having a physical body makes you vulnerable to all sorts of pain from the moment of birth until you die. Throughout your life you endure pain and suffering: your first teeth come in and tear through your gums, you bump your head or hit your knees while learning to walk, you suffer through a variety of childhood diseases, not to mention random head-aches, stomach upsets, muscle pains, and more. In addition you go through countless non-physical hurts: the death of a loved one, the break-up with your first lover, the loss of a friend or life partner, the rejection and shaming by peers, and all the mind-wrecking existential worries and fears.

Nothing hurts more than your own self-attack

"Only my condemnation injures me."
A Course In Miracles

One of your greatest fears in life is being hurt, especially by another human being. You are anxious about not being welcomed or wanted. You avoid situations in which another might attack you, criticize you, make you wrong, judge you, or reject you. But what you may not realize is that the greatest hurt you endure over the course your life is not caused by another person or distressing circumstances. The deepest wounding in your life comes from yourself. Nothing will ever hurt you more and produce more pain than the way you attack, criticize, judge, condemn, reject, punish, and abandon yourself. Whenever you are hurt, feel scared, or experience a defeat, what you need the most in such moments is to feel protected, taken care of, and loved. Yet, you usually do the exact opposite! You attack yourself. You criticize and judge yourself. You blame, shame, and make yourself wrong for being who you are and for being in this painful situation in the first place. Then you walk away and abandon this judged, rejected, despised, and essentially unloved part of you. And what remains hidden away in the depth of your subconscious bodymind is repressed pain, in the shape of another unloved *shadow patch*.

Whatever you attack, reject, and repress begins to hurt and form a shadow patch inside your bodymind that blocks the rays of your Inner Sun.

The "happiness-killer" — your inner critic

The inner critic is the *happiness-killer* in your life. Every time the inner critic is attacking, criticizing, and judging the unwanted aspects and experiences of yourself, you hurt yourself. Through self-attack the inner critic inflicts acute pain on you. Besides the acute pain, secondary or chronic pain is also created. This chronic pain is the direct result of all these repressed little hurts that keep accumulating. Over the years this inner war takes its toll on you. It erodes your sense of self-worth and undermines your self-confidence. It impacts your bodymind by using up enormous quantities of your vital energy to sustain the self-attacks and hold down all these rejected parts of yourself. This inner stress caused by your inner critic and its ideal self-demands that say how you *should be* and how you *shouldn't be* can produce a multitude of psychosomatic symptoms. Chronic tension, shallow breathing, fatigue, hypersensitivity, irritation, bad sleep, nightmares, avoidance of intimacy, absent-mindedness, and addictions— as well as all sorts of little and big aches, including serious illnesses—can result. The inner critic's self-attack in the name of establishing your ideal self has the potential to turn your inner world into a dark place. This is the work of the inner critic, the *false savior* in you that is in actual fact the real happiness-killer.

Eva Broch-Pierrakos expresses this beautifully in a paragraph from one of her lectures called the *Idealized Self-Image*, "Since the standards and dictates of the Idealized Self are impossible to realize, yet never giving up the attempt, you keep and cultivate within yourself an inner tyranny of the worst order. But since you do not realize the impossibility of being as perfect as your Idealized Self demands, you never give up whipping yourself, castigating yourself, and feeling yourself a complete failure whenever it is proven that you cannot do so. The sense of abject worthlessness comes over you whenever you fall short of these fantastic demands and engulfs you in misery." [14]

THE GREATER THE THREAT — THE GREATER THE NEED FOR SAFETY

The louder, the more authoritarian, and demanding the voice of your inner critic the more terrifying and existentially threatening appears the inner or outer situation to be. The harsher the self-attack the greater is your inner child's need for safety.

Fully understanding the relationship between the inner critic and the inner child enables you to be more compassionate with yourself, especially while the inner critic's negative self-talk is going on inside your head. The more often you remind yourself that the inner critic is the internalized parental voice that is really trying to protect the inner child, the easier it will be to change tracks and relate to yourself in a more kindhearted way once you notice the self-attack. In such a moment you might say to yourself, "Oh, my inner child feels terrified. She/he is in need of more safety."

Occasionally you might even be able to smile at yourself when the tyrannical voice of your inner critic resounds. What helps me is simply to bring awareness to myself by saying, "Oh, my inner child feels terrified." Then, as a second step, I ask myself, "What would make my inner child more safe right now?" These two steps alone usually take the wind right out of the sails of the inner critic and make the little boy calm down immediately.

The bottom line is: whenever your inner critic attacks, some part of you feels terrified and needs safety. You can call this part your inner child, *Little Jane, Little Tom* or your *Inner Animal*, whatever you like. These terms like inner critic or inner child are simply terms to give names for aspects and processes within your bodymind. You can use my terms or a term that you resonate with. What counts is that you choose a name that makes you feel more compassionate towards the *scared part* in you and calls forth the loving parent or caretaker in you.

**"If there is no enemy within,
the enemy outside can do you no harm."**
African Proverb

IT'S YOUR JOB TO LOVE YOUR INNER CHILD!

The upset, scared, hurt and suffering inner child in you needs to be consciously recognized, reassured, looked after, and loved. As adults, we tend to either ignore or repress these scared and needy parts, or to delegate them to someone else to take care of, for example, a lover, life partner, friend, doctor, psychiatrist, therapist, healer, or whoever. But the truth is nobody else can fully take care of your inner child with all its needy, neglected, and immature aspects. This is your job. The inner child belongs to you and it is your assignment to watch over your inner kid and to re-parent it. Your parents did the best they could, whether you think it was good enough or not does not really matter. If you want to become a mature, integrated, and loving human being then it is your task to parent—*to mother and father*— your inner child. To love it!

LOVING YOURSELF IS THE SOLUTION

The good news is you can learn to love yourself! I know this from my own experience since I truly hated myself and often suffered from intense *self-loathing-attacks*, especially in my early childhood and as a teenager. I hated my body, the way I looked, and how I felt emotionally. Often I just felt miserable and depressed without any obvious external reasons. To me it felt as if a dark cloud hovered over my head nearly all the time. No matter what I did, it just would not go away. At the time I was sure that if only I could get rid of my emotional body, I would no longer have to suffer. Secretly I wished that I could take a knife, stab my emotional body, cut it out of my energy field, and bury it somewhere in the garden. Well, later through my personal research and education in body-centered psychotherapy, somatic education, energy healing, and yoga, I finally discovered that every dark cloud—no matter the density of its emotional content—gradually transforms and dissolves into blue sky. The key is: I have to choose to relate to it in a conscious and loving way.

**Loving yourself frees you from the pain caused by
the inner critic and awakens the inner lover in you, which is
the foundation to love yourself & another/others as well.**

If you are ready to learn the nuts and bolts of the Art of Selflove, then let's move on to Part Two of this book.

"Selflove Begins With You"

CHAPTER 4

"Waking Up" - Self-Awareness & the Birth of Selflove

"To the person who watches, everything reveals itself."
Italian Proverb

ABOVE the entrance of the Temple of Apollo where the Oracle of Delphi resided in ancient Greece the words *Gnothi Seauton* are inscribed in golden letters. This translates into English as *Know Thyself*—a potent directive, and one you will discover is essential to the Art of Selflove.

The first step in building a conscious and loving relationship with yourself is to become aware. Self-awareness is the basis of self-exploration and self-discovery, which automatically leads to a greater comprehension of yourself. What you explore you begin to understand as it reveals its deeper nature to you. Self-awareness, then, is the foundation on which you can build a solid understanding of who you truly are and thereby reap the benefits of "know thyself" as your essence is revealed ever more fully.

You approach this in much the same way as you would a foreign culture that you want to understand. Upon arriving in an alien country you begin to investigate by observing the people, studying their behavior, and learning their language. You have to immerse yourself in their way of life in order to get to know them. Eventually you will begin to comprehend what the people are saying, why they do what they do, what they value, what they strive for, and what they view as important goals. What seemed very strange in the beginning gradually becomes familiar to you.

**"Knowing others is wisdom –
Knowing yourself is enlightenment."**
Lao Tse

The very same is true when you begin to explore your inner life. If you want to know and understand yourself, you have to become observant. This is very different from the type of nervous self-consciousness that is evidenced so often in people's behavior. Self-awareness is quite different in quality than self-consciousness. A self-aware person is characterized by curiosity and interest, whereas someone who is self-conscious is agitated and overly concerned with his or her image.

Self-awareness frees you from the spell of self-consciousness and opens the door to Selflove. Now, you might wonder: "What is that I need to become aware of in myself? What exactly do I bring my awareness to?"

ALL YOU'VE EVER GOT IS YOUR AWARENESS

The only *thing* you will ever have is your own awareness, and it is through the agency of your awareness that you consciously encounter your inner and outer world. What you are aware of becomes your experience and therefore becomes part of your reality. Essentially all you can ever relate to with your awareness is your here and now experience. Said another way, where you focus your awareness determines what you will experience. You might say, "I've got a body, a lover or a life partner, a family, a car, a job, an apartment or a house, etc." You are right. You've got all that. All these things are real. They exist and are part of your life. Fundamentally, everything that you notice in your life is simply an experience that you register through your awareness.

**Through your awareness you become conscious
of your here and now experience.**

The whole exterior world of nature, people, objects, plants, and animals are perceived through your sense organs: sight, hearing, touch, smell, and taste.

These sense perceptions allow you to experience the outer world. Additionally, you have an interior world that you experience through dreams, imagination, concepts, ideas, and fantasies. Any experience you have is either directly or indirectly stimulated by your exterior or interior world. If you were suddenly cut off from all of your five senses then you would no longer be able to perceive the outer world. You would feel as though you had lost everything that was ever a part of you *out there*. The external world with all the people, possessions and things that are so dear to you would still exist for everyone else, but they would vanish for you. Unable to bring your awareness to the outer world, you no longer perceive it. This is exactly what happens while you are in a deep sleep or a coma. The outer world is *lost* to you. It no longer exists because you can no longer register sense impressions from the exterior world.

The only way you can ever relate to yourself, to your loved ones,
to your fellow human beings and your environment,
is by relating to your experience of them in the here & now.

Have you ever wondered what it is inside of you that is aware of your experience?

THE INNER OBSERVER

"The movements within the individual consciousness can only
be perceived by that which witnesses them, the fundamental
background of root-consciousness, which is Stillness, the Self."
Patanjali - Yoga Sutras

Your individual consciousness is characterized by an *inner observer* that simply witnesses and perceives *what is*. This conscious *I* has one main function: to be aware and to notice your here and now experience. You can imagine the inner observer as an eye that has a wide, expansive view and can see what you are experiencing from a detached, big-picture perspective. I call the inner observer the *Big Eye* to symbolize this wider viewpoint. From this central aspect of your conscious personality "you" are not identified with any of your experiences. It is the inner observer that is aware and allows you to become conscious of your here and now experience in a completely open, non-attached, and non-judgmental way.

The inner observer is the *Big Eye*, the inner awareness in you that is fully conscious of all of your experiences.

Throughout this book I will often refer to the inner observer to reinforce the importance of developing self-awareness in order to cultivate the Art of Selflove. At this point it might be helpful to know that every time you practice the Welcoming-Process—the central Selflove-method that you will learn in Part Three —you automatically strengthen the inner observer as well.

You always have
the option to step
intentionally into
the Inner Observer,
the "Big Eye".

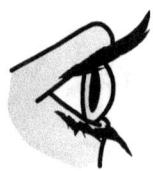

The "Big Eye"
...is aware of the
content of your here &
now experience.

The content of experience

Have you ever consciously explored your experience to see what it is made of? Everything that happens to you consists of specific elements that I refer to as the *content of experience*. This is an important expression that I will use over and over to emphasize that any experience is made up of specific content that can be clearly identified and described in words. The purpose of differentiating between the various types of content is to support you in centering yourself in the inner observer. Let's lay the groundwork by naming each category and establishing a descriptive language.

The 5 Elements of Experience

In order to distinguish between the various contents of human experience, I have delineated five basic categories, called the *5 Elements of Experience*. Every experience, regardless of its content, consists of one or more of these fundamental elements.

The 5 Elements of Experience are as follows:

1. Body-sensations & sense perceptions
2. Needs & desires
3. Emotions & feelings
4. Thoughts, ideas, & concepts
5. Images, symbols, dreams, fantasies, stories, & memories

The purpose of this list is to help you become aware of *what the actual content of your experience is* and thus support the development of your inner observer.

THE FLOWER OF EXPERIENCE

The *Flower of Experience* is a simple metaphor that will help you understand how the various elements of experience are related to your inner observer. Each flower petal stands for one element of experience. In the middle of the flower you see the inner observer that is fully aware of each of the 5 Elements of Experience. Symbolically speaking, the inner observer is the stem and the bud out of which the five petals grow. Therefore the inner observer is much more than the petals with their various experiences. The job of your inner observer is to remain in a centered state of observation —to remain neutral and unaffected by the actual content of experience. The picture of the Flower of Experience shows the center position that the inner observer ideally holds while observing the 5 Elements of Experience.

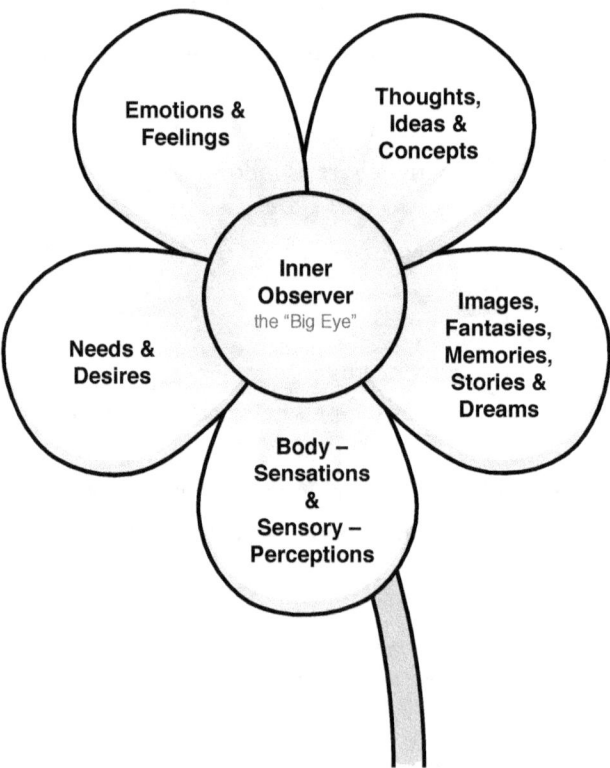

Let's look at each of the 5 Elements of Experience in more detail.

Body-sensations

Perhaps you've heard it said that human beings become *human doings* in a society that urges us to focus on achievement above all else while placing little, if any, emphasis on quiet introspection. The tendency to focus on the external world and disregard the physical body has become more and more prevalent in our technological age. I see the effect of this quite often in my private practice. As a somatic[4] (body-centered) therapist, my job is to guide and assist people as they build a perceptual bridge so they can "land" in their physicality.

Being out of touch with your body and physical sensations is a real loss because your body can give you clear information about the overall state of your bodymind. In other words, your body speaks to you in the language of sensation and it is fluent as to what your needs are in any given moment. *Body-sensations[5]* as well as body gestures are part of the language repertoire of the subconscious. Therefore, the most natural way for you to get to know your subconscious mind is to become aware of body-sensations. For example, when you start feeling tense in a certain situation, your subconscious is communicating that it feels insecure and somewhat threatened, and is in need of security. If, on the other hand, your body begins to relax and to breathe more deeply, then the subconscious lets you know that it feels reassured and everything is okay. Subconscious, intuitive messages are transmitted in the form of distinct body-sensations. By reading this book and by practicing the Welcoming-Process you will get very familiar with a wide range of body-sensations. Continue to pay attention and, over time, you will be able to translate their underlying or deeper message.

Many people confuse body-sensations with emotions and feelings or think that these two are one and the same. This work will help you differentiate between the two so that you can listen to your inner life with a keen and sensitive ear.

---

[4] *Soma* is a Greek term which refers to the living body experienced from within; rather than the physical body that is looked at from the outside, from another person's perspective. In Somatic Education the goal is to assist the client in becoming aware of his own body, to experience it from within, by clearly sensing the sensations in one's body (i.e. body-sensations).

[5] A body-sensation is the sensation you feel in your physical body. Becoming aware of your body-sensations is the foundation to *Notice the Bodyshift*, which is the 3rd Step of the Welcoming-Process, the central method to cultivate the Art of Selflove. On the next page you will find a list of the various types of body-sensations.

VARIOUS TYPES OF BODY-SENSATIONS

The list below gives examples of various types of body-sensations. It is offered as a primer, rather than an exhaustive list; use it to begin your discovery process and distinguish the variety of ways your body lets you know what is happening just below the surface of your awareness.

- Breathing: movements in your belly and/or chest area in the form of inhalation and exhalation
- Muscle tone: tension/relaxation, such as hard, tight, firm, soft, supple, elastic, etc.
- Movement sensations: tingling, shaking, streaming, flowing, pulsing, stinging, pushing, calming or slowing down, speeding up, etc.
- Temperature sensations: warm, cold, lukewarm, cool, fiery, icy, etc.
- Weight sensation: light/heavy
- Sensation of space: open, closed, wide, tight, full, empty, solid, dispersed, etc.
- Sensation of presence: you feel present in your body—grounded, rooted, centered, connected, etc.
- Body sounds: gurgling, grumbling, whistling, etc.

QUESTIONS TO IDENTIFY YOUR BODY-SENSATIONS:

1. What do you sense in your body right now?
2. Where do you sense it in your body?
3. What type of body-sensation is it?
4. What is the name or word that describes this body-sensation in the most accurate way?

When you find the right word for a certain body-sensation, you will feel an inner nudge or feeling of: "Yes, that resonates." This is your body's way of confirming that you've hit on an accurate description. Once you learn to consciously sense the different types of body-sensations, to precisely describe and name them, you will have made a giant leap in gaining more self-awareness.

Sensory-perceptions

Sensory-perceptions include all the impressions that come from the external world that you register or perceive through one or more of your five physical senses. They consist of sight or vision coming from your eyes, hearing from your ears, smell from your nose, taste from your tongue, and touch from your skin. Any uncensored perception that you receive directly from one of the external sensory channels of your body is called a sensory-perception. For example: you see a silver spoon, smell camphor, sense the sweat running down your brow, hear a loud noise, taste a bitter food, etc. Since you are very familiar with your five physical senses, you will find this element of experience easy to identify.

Although sensory-perceptions and body-sensations are distinctly different, I have—for the sake of simplicity—put body-sensations and sensory-perceptions into the same category or element of experience. To distinguish between the two is very simple: if you register an experience through one of your five senses, it is a sensory-perception, whereas a physical sensation that emerges from within your body is a body-sensation. Knowing the difference between the two will help you develop awareness of your body-sensation since these tend to go unnoticed by many of us.

Needs & desires

A need is a fundamental, biological drive that first of all wants to be consciously recognized and secondly, if possible, to be satisfied.

How do you know that you are hungry or thirsty? How do you know that you have a need? Your body tells you. To be more precise: your body nudges you very subtly. (This category overlaps to some degree with body-sensation.)

Have you ever really sat with your hunger or thirst long enough to become intimately aware of the exact sensations that signal you when it is time to eat or take a drink? Could you describe these in detail? Next time when you are hungry or thirsty, take a moment and consciously explore what you sense in your body. This is a powerful way to make a previously unconscious body signal more conscious.

Becoming aware of your body-sensations & body signals
is the way to get to know your needs.

All your basic needs, including your inner urges, are rooted in your biology. They are instinctual by nature and thus controlled by your subconscious mind. You cannot make yourself hungry or thirsty when you are not because hunger and thirst are involuntary, subconscious manifestations of your bodymind. Your body speaks to you through body-sensations. The various body-sensa-tions inform you about your need for safety, food, movement, rest, sexuality, boundaries, alone time, closeness, the right touch, or the appropriate distance between you and another person. Your body-sensations are innately intelligent signals of your body. Paying attention to your body-sensations is a direct way to develop your intuition and to access the intelligence of your subconscious mind that supports you in living a more harmonious life.

Where you draw the line between a need and a desire is your personal choice and does not really matter since they belong to the same element of experience.

The American Psychologist Abraham Maslow*4 researched the lives of successful and influential people and eventually developed his *Theory of Human Motivation*. He discovered that throughout the world all human beings have the same basic needs. Maslow organized the human needs into five categories; these have become known as *Maslow's Hierarchy of Needs*. These 5 categories build on each other like the different levels of a pyramid stacked according to importance.

At the bottom of the pyramid are the basic survival needs of the body: breathing, nourishment, sleep, sex, and everything that sustains us at the level of our physiology. The second level deals with the need for safety and security in the physical, psychological, and material realm. The third or middle level represents the need for loving relationships and social belonging in the form of partnership, family, friends, and communal participation, which gener-ally translates as what you do for work. The fourth level relates to the need for esteem and social recognition; this includes self-esteem, self-confidence, achievements, respect of others, status, and influence. These four lower levels are associated with the needs of the body. Just as it is true for animals, human beings have an instinctual drive to satisfy the needs of their bodies.

At the highest level, the capstone of the pyramid represents our built-in need for self-actualization. This includes developing our abilities, forming ethical standards, expressing talents, as well as developing essential qualities such as creativity, compassion, honesty, patience, etc. The pursuit of needs on the top level is geared towards the search for happiness and the realization of one's full potential. Maslow labeled this top level *growth needs* or *being values*; they are non-physical, psychological, and spiritual needs that all human beings share once the lower needs are met. I think of these *higher needs* as desires because they go beyond the purely instinctual level.

By natural law, the higher needs or desires only arise when the lower needs are satisfied. In other words, whenever a lower need is not sufficiently met, your attention automatically focuses on satisfying it. Then and only then is your attention free to pursue the higher order needs.

EMOTIONS & FEELINGS

Every human being experiences a vast spectrum of emotions and feelings. According to psychologist Robert Plutchik's *Psychoevolutionary Theory of Emotion*5, there are eight primary emotions: anger, fear, sadness, disgust, surprise, curiosity, acceptance, and joy. His theory asserts that these emotions have their root in our biology and actually have survival value. Of course, we experience many more shades and tones of emotion than just these basic eight, and these could be enumerated in an almost endless list. Life is full of moments that are colored by insecurity, grief, loneliness, longing, lust, awe, hate, bitterness, jealousy, self-pity, pride, melancholy, worry, guilt, resent-ment, boredom, excitement, shyness, frustration, and... the list goes on and on. All emotions and feelings are essentially related to the eight basic emotions to some degree.

Whether you call an emotional experience an emotion or a feeling is your personal choice. Some people make a distinction between the two, but for the purpose of this work what matters is the clear distinction between body-sensations and emotions & feelings—the first stands for body-centered signals and sensations and the latter for emotional, feeling experiences—because this will help you zero in when you begin doing the Welcoming-Process.

THOUGHTS, IDEAS & CONCEPTS

Any experience that finds you thinking, reflecting, analyzing, questioning, playing with ideas, or even passively ruminating over familiar, mindless thoughts falls into this category. The element of experience—*thoughts, ideas & concepts*—can also include multi-faceted aspects of thinking such as dialectic, inquiry, insight, and arriving at a deeper understanding. If you analyze a specific thought in more detail, you might discover that it is really a statement, a judgment, an opinion, an assumption, a belief, or a conviction, just to name a few. For our objective, it is enough to identify your experience as a thought and to fit it into the category of thoughts, ideas & concepts.

IMAGES, FANTASIES, MEMORIES, STORIES & DREAMS

The element of experience of *images, fantasies, memories, stories & dreams* contains all experiences that come in the form of pictures, movie-like scenes, or symbols. If you observe your content of experience and recognize that it is of a visual quality then you know that it falls in this category. Since the element of experience of thoughts, ideas & concepts is so closely related with the one of images, fantasies, memories, stories & dreams you decide which one of the two feels more appropriate.

INVITATION TO IDENTIFY THE 5 ELEMENTS OF EXPERIENCE

Below you will find a list of 20 statements. After you read each state-ment ask yourself, "Which category of the 5 Elements of Experience does this content fit into?" It is good to mention that this exercise is not a test; it is a matter of choice. There is no right or wrong answer. How you identify a content of experience is subjective and individual. You might catego-rize a certain content of experience as a need & desire, whereas someone else might classify it as an emotion & feeling. From your point of view some of the statements might even fit into two or more categories. Simply choose the category that you resonate with the most and make sure that you know why you identify a certain content of experience the way you do. The basic guide-line is: your choice is the right one.

Once you have named the element of experience, write your answer down next to each statement. You can also look at the illustration of the Flower of

Experience on page 58, in order to assist you in making your choice. Have fun identifying each of the following 20 statements!

1. I feel exhausted.
2. I want the stock market to go up.
3. I cannot let it go.
4. I can picture the situation.
5. My body feels tight.
6. I have a bitter taste in my mouth.
7. I am afraid that I will end up living alone.
8. I long to live a more adventurous life.
9. My muscles are sore.
10. I don't care about being the best.
11. I feel tension in my belly.
12. I remember the operation.
13. I have more courage.
14. He is insensitive to other people's feelings.
15. I dream of a house in the countryside.
16. I feel happy.
17. I hear a high-pitched sound.
18. I feel so angry I could punch him.
19. My whole body feels more grounded, more present.
20. I can see very clearly how my room looked like when I was a teenager.

WHAT IS THE PURPOSE OF DIFFERENTIATING YOUR CONTENT OF EXPERIENCE?

The purpose of analyzing and identifying the content of your experience is to assist you in cultivating your awareness of the inner observer. The inner observer, or Big Eye, is key in becoming aware of your here and now experience and thus in developing your self-awareness, which is the first step in the Art of Selflove.

Once you are familiar with the Welcoming-Process, you will see how identifying the elements of experience will help you save time as you are taking yourself through the process.

"BEING AWARE OR UNAWARE" - THIS IS THE QUESTION

Every time you have an experience, you have a choice. Either you stay aware of your experience and consciously observe it as it is, or you *lose yourself* in the actual content of your experience and become completely identified with it. The two diagrams below will help you understand these two scenarios in more detail.

CENTEREDNESS: THE PERSPECTIVE OF THE INNER OBSERVER

The Inner Observer

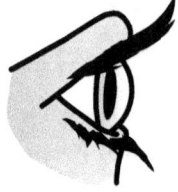

The Content of Experience

The "Big Eye"
...is aware of...
...is conscious of...
...perceives...

The Big Eye represents the inner observer—the conscious "I" in you that sees and recognizes *what is*. The above diagram shows that the Big Eye or the inner observer always stays *outside* of your experience, in a somewhat distant position. This enables you to remain centered in the inner observer, and therefore to consciously witness the actual content of your experience. It is important to remember that the inner observer never gets swallowed up by the content of your experience and therefore does not become identified with the experience, no matter what the actual content is. It simply witnesses, perceives, and notices what you experience in a neutral and detached mode.

The inner observer, the Big Eye states,
"I am aware", or "I am conscious of..."

IDENTIFICATION: "BEING LOST IN YOUR EXPERIENCE"

If you are no longer conscious of the inner observer, you become your *little-i*, which is totally *lost in the cloud of experience* and thus completely identified with its content. The diagram below gives you a graphic representation of this situation:

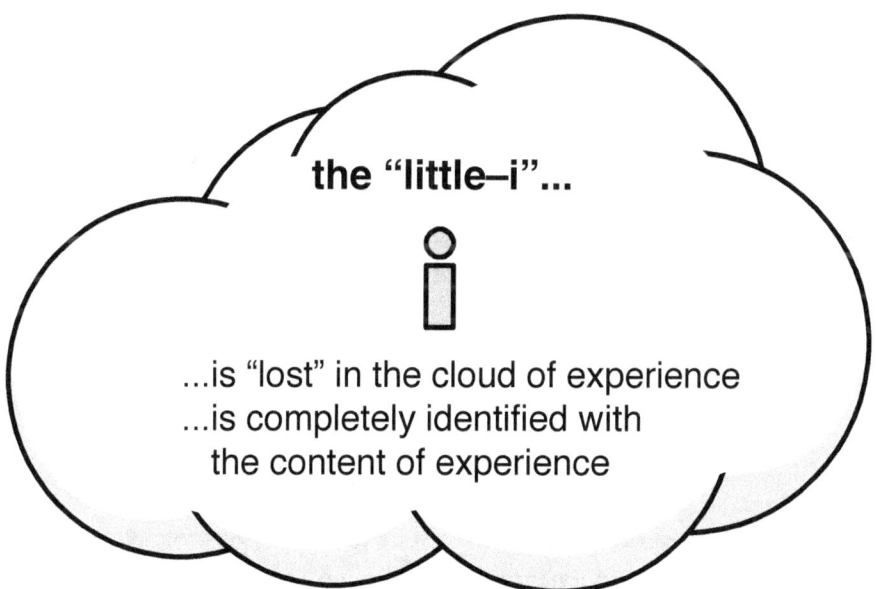

the "little–i"...

...is "lost" in the cloud of experience
...is completely identified with
the content of experience

If you do not practice self-observation, you will be completely immersed in your own experience throughout your life. This means you are fully consumed by the drama of your life, and out of touch with your inner observer. Each time you are fully engrossed in your experience, you, automatically become your *little-i*. The little-i is the part in you that is fully identified with the content of your experience and believes what you experience is who you are. This misidentification (who you are is much more than what you experience in any moment) is the reason why the little-i has no capacity to observe the actual content of your experience.

Marshall Govindan and Jan Ahlund point out in their book, *Kriya Yoga: Insights Along the Path*, how we habitually mistake the content of our experience for who we truly are: "...we confuse the Self with the non-Self, the permanent with the impermanent."... "In other words egoism is the habit of identifying with what we are not, the body-mind personality, the instrument of cognition, as well as thoughts, sensations, and emotions. We fail to recognize that they are objects, merely reflections of our awareness."[6]

Have you ever gotten so completely caught up in a gripping movie that you were no longer aware of the fact that you are sitting in a movie theatre? You become so fully identified with the story, the historical setting, and the characters in the film, especially with the main character. You live in them and they live in you. Even your physiology responds to what is occurring on screen as though it is actually happening to you. The story and the characters move you so deeply, they fully absorb your attention and become *your drama* for that period of time. It is as if you died, reincarnated, and took on a new personality called Luke Skywalker, Indiana Jones, Lara Croft, Harry Potter, Frodo Baggins, or whatever character you temporarily identify with. And then the lights come up and the drama is over. In exactly the same way, we get wrapped up in the various experiences of our own lives.

THE NATURE OF THE little-i

The little-i is always in a reactive mode because it gets totally caught up in the content of your experience. Since it has no access to the inner observer and no capacity to self-reflect, it cannot stand back, observe, and analyze your here and now experience. It reacts impulsively in predictable and habitual ways. If the little-i is in danger, it gets scared and tries to protect itself by either attacking the source of the threat or by running away from it. If, on the other hand, the experience is enjoyable and satisfying, the little-i gets attached or even addicted to the source of pleasure. The little-i takes every experience very personally for it looks at the world through a filter that constantly refers back to itself. Its refrain is a never ending song and dance of *i, me & mine*. If it gets satisfaction or receives praise, it feels great and on top of the world—for a time. When it gets even the slightest form of criticism or is no longer the center of attention it feels instantly hurt and upset. The little-i lays at the root of all egotism and lack of consideration for others, since it is completely *i-centered & i*-absorbed.*

*(see the Reaction Pattern of the little-i in Chapter 5 on page 82.)

WEATHER PATTERNS IN A LIMITLESS SKY

You are much more than your experience. This is true for you, me, and everyone; we are always much more than the content of our experience. You are not your body-sensations, needs, desires, emotions, feelings, thoughts, ideas, concepts, images, fantasies, memories, stories & dreams. The various types of experiences are like clouds produced by constantly changing weather patterns in the atmosphere. You are more like the limitless sky that gives birth to the weather itself. Even though you continuously identify yourself with the ever-changing weather conditions of your experiential world, who you truly are is much more than that. The little-i is so completely engrossed and entangled in its content of experience that it believes experience is who it is. If the experience is sadness or anger, the little-i says, "i am sad." or "i am angry."

What you've got is not who you are.
Who you are is not what you've got.

The inner observer or Big Eye in you is never identified with the content of any experience. It can never be sad or angry; it simply perceives, "I am aware of sadness." or "I notice some anger." The nature of the inner observer is to remain in an entirely neutral and centered position from which all experi-ences—independent of their content—are witnessed.

"We are not our emotions, not our desires, nor our thoughts.
We are not our three bodies, but something far greater."
Panayota Theotoki-Atteshli

DEATH OF THE little-i & AWAKENING OF THE INNER OBSERVER

When you go through a major personal crisis such as the loss of a loved one, your little-i becomes terrified that the pain of separation will destroy it. This delusion of the little-i can be so convincing that you feel as if you will not survive. But in reality the inner observer can never be uprooted by any experience, since it always remains fully centered in the Self.

And in fact, for many people, when the little-i gets so shaken that it can no longer masquerade as the psyche's foundation, the larger Self reveals itself with a searing clarity that changes you forever.

Such a crossroads moment happened to me in 2002. My wife had made it clear to me that she wanted to have a child but I felt intense fear and resistance each time she brought up the subject. I knew she expected a yes or no answer in the very near future, and I knew that I might lose her if I could not agree with what she wanted. So I decided to travel to Asia where I could spend some time alone and give myself space to see how I really felt about having a child.

From this point on the story will be told in the present tense, since the immediacy and intensity of this incident is still so vivid in my memory it is as if it is happening right now.

Three months pass and I am returning to her with complete clarity on how I feel about stepping into fatherhood. We go for a walk along the lake where we live, and when we arrive at our favorite spot, she asks, "Frank, do you want a child with me?" I know this is the moment of truth that I have dreaded so much. Nonetheless, I know that I have to tell her my truth, "I don't feel ready to have a child with you." She looks into my eyes. Hers are filled with sadness as she says, "Then, our marriage is over." I hear these words and feel as if an axe is plunging right through me; it splits me apart from top to bottom. I burst into tears and my whole body is shaking and trembling from all the emotions and feelings that break loose in me. I am no longer crying, the moment is *crying me*. The pain is excruciating, beyond words. I feel like a baby that has just lost his mother. All I can do is to give in to the bawling and sobbing that comes out of the center of my body. In between the up-welling waves of emotion, I find myself gasping for air. It is as if I am going through the agony of dying. Yet, while all of this is happening, a part of me remains completely calm and simply watches the whole process. This neutral observer just witnesses what is going on. It notices all these intense emotions as if they were clouds that pass by in front of a blue sky. Most of me is absorbed in the emotional hurt of just having lost my wife, and yet this presence just observes in an absolutely detached manner. As I reach the climax of this tearing pain that seems to rip me apart, I see an image of a tree whose trunk is split down in the middle. That's when the searing realization comes: I see that there is a point where no tree and no root can be split any further because all trees and all roots have their origin in this place. I realize, "Right from here emerges everything and right here everything is whole and one." In that moment, I know from deep inside that everything is good just as it is and that I will survive the separation from my wife, no matter what I will have to go through in the process.

WHO AM I?

"You are an unlimited being. You always were and you always will be, you have no choice in that. Your only choice is to identify with your unlimited beingness or to identify with your self-imposed limitations."
Lester Levenson

The question, "Who am I?" is as old as humanity. Nobody can answer this question in a satisfactory way, because who you truly are is beyond any intellectual concept or rational comprehension. To find out who you are is a process of discovery that leads you to the inner experience and realization of your very Self. To walk this path of self-realization requires self-awareness which brings about the clear distinction between the little-i and the inner observer in you. Through the consistent practice of self-awareness and self-observation you keep refining your perception, and this in turn allows you to gain ever-deeper insights into your human nature—the nature of your body, your emotions, your mind, and the way you relate to yourself and others. Ever more often you will go beyond the layers of your mask and your shadow self and enter the sphere of your Divine Self, the source of love and happiness within you.

No self-awareness—No Selflove

When you are fully absorbed in the content of your experience (as illustrated in the diagram on Identification, page 67) you are no longer in touch with the inner observer. Self-awareness is lost as well. Therefore, if you are unaware of your here and now experience, you can no longer relate to the content of your experience in a conscious and loving way. This insight leads us to the simple rule: No self-awareness—No Selflove. Now, it becomes obvious why self-awareness is the 1st step of the Art of Selflove.

Self-awareness is self-empowerment

Self-awareness empowers you to choose how you want to relate to yourself.

Self-awareness is self-empowerment because it provides you with the choice of how you want to relate to yourself, and, in particular, to your experience. Each time you become aware of the actual content of your here and now experience you empower yourself since you center yourself in the inner observer—the foundation of all conscious choice. Self-awareness and freedom of choice are the natural gifts that you receive from the inner observer.

The 1ˢᵀ step of the Art Selflove

The Inner Observer

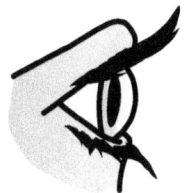

The Content of Experience

The "Big Eye"
...is aware of...
...is conscious of...
...perceives...

Consciously making contact with the content of your here & now experience represents the 1ˢᵗ step of the Art of Selflove.

Once you are aware of the content of your experience, you are ready for the 2ⁿᵈ step of the Art of Selflove: choice of attitude, the subject of the next chapter.

CHAPTER 5

Selflove is a Choice

**"The greatest discovery of any generation is that a human being
can alter his life by altering his attitude."**
William James

YOUR EXPERIENCE IS AS IT IS

LIFE *just is.* Grass is green. The sky is blue. Blood is red. Likewise, your experience just is as it is. If you feel happy, you feel happy. If you feel angry, you feel angry. If you have a craving for chocolate, you have a craving for chocolate. If your tummy hurts, your tummy hurts. If you would like to do more sports, you would like to do more sports. If you dream of having a beautiful home, you dream of having a beautiful home. Whatever the content of your experience is, this is your experience. Life is as it is and your experience is as it is.

This simple truth cannot be emphasized enough. Most of the time you don't perceive your experience *as it is* because you are wrapped up in the habit of evaluating the contents of your experience. Moreover, you are largely unaware that you are doing so. Essentially there is just experience—your here and now experience, your subjective reality in the present moment. Whether you like your current experience or not, whether you call it good or bad, positive or negative is your call. You have exclusive rights when it comes to evaluating your experience.

"There is nothing either good or bad but thinking makes it so."
William Shakespeare

THE 4 BASIC WANTS OF THE little-i

The little-i evaluates and judges every experience based on four fundamental objectives, which I refer to as the *4 Basic Wants**. They are:

---

1. **The want to be/feel safe**
2. **The want to be/feel loved**
3. **The want to be/feel satisfied**
4. **The want to be/feel in control**

The little-i is instinctively programmed to chase after and satisfy these 4 Basic Wants. It has no choice about that. Its job description reads: scan for, detect, and pursue any experience that promises to fulfill any one of these 4 Basic Wants. Most of the time your feelings, your thinking, and your imagination are directly, or indirectly, involved in pursuing a basic want. Shortly after the little-i has satisfied one want, it instantly leaps into the next pursuit.

If you take a moment and analyze your interactions with other people you will discover that the motivation behind what you do is influenced by one of the 4 Basic Wants. Everything you do in an unconscious, habitual, and reactive mode is determined by the 4 Basic Wants.

* With sincere appreciation I would like to acknowledge the fact that my concept of the "4 Basic Wants of the little-i" was inspired by Lester Levenson, the founder of the Sedona Method®. Any similarities between my work, the Welcoming- Process™, and the Sedona Method® are unintentional.

WHAT MAKES A "GOOD" OR A "BAD" EXPERIENCE?

Any experience that satisfies a basic want is a *good* experience and any experience that doesn't is a *bad* one.

The little-i is intimately connected with what is often called the *reptilian brain*, the biologically anchored survival system located in the brain stem and the cerebellum that automatically checks out every experience to see if it satisfies one of the 4 Basic Wants. Every experience that fulfills one of the 4 Basic Wants is judged as *good* or *positive* and every experience that does not is *bad* or *negative.* Your little-i is in love with the good/positive experiences and at war with the bad/negative ones.

The little-i naturally supports and goes after the so-called good or positive experiences because they fulfill a basic want. The more an actual experience satisfies any of the 4 Basic Wants the more attractive and more positive it is for the little-i. An experience that makes you feel safe, appreciated or loved, and additionally gives you a sense of satisfaction and control fulfills all 4 Basic Wants. It will be rated as a top experience. Your little-i relishes such experiences and will compel you to pursue them intensely and as often as possible, often at great expense. You will find yourself attached or even addicted to activities that profoundly satisfy your basic wants.

I can give you a number of examples, such as eating your favorite meal, spending all day in bed with your lover, or having a stimulating conversation with your best friend, however, you will gain more self-awareness by looking for yourself at how you gratify your 4 Basic Wants on a day to day basis.

What satisfies the 4 Basic Wants in your life?

The following questions are an invitation to find out where and how in your life you try to satisfy your 4 Basic Wants. Simply by answering the following questions you will gain insight into your behavior and begin to recognize the motivation behind your daily activities.

1) Ask yourself the following questions and write them down in your personal notebook:

- How do you spend most of your energy?
- What do you enjoy doing the most in your free time?
- What would you like to have more time for?
- What are you fond of doing when you are alone?
- What do you love to do with your partner, your best friend, and your family members?
- When you have extra money, what do you spend it on?
- What are you willing to save money for?
- If you had lots of money what would you spend it on?
- What experiences leave the lingering feeling: *I can never get enough!*

- What makes you feel the most alive?

2) Now go back to the answers you wrote to the questions above and consider each response, asking yourself these two questions:

- Which of the 4 Basic Wants does it fulfill?
- How does it fulfill this basic want in you?

Your answers will give you a clear understanding of how these 4 Basic Wants influence your behavior and the way you live.

THE THREE SURVIVAL RESPONSES

Negative or so-called bad experiences, always run contrary to at least one of the 4 Basic Wants. Since these wants are directly linked with your survival needs, this opposition activates aversion and resistance within the little-i. The experience will register in you as uncomfortable, disturbing, or painful, and the little-i will respond with resistance and aversion. Every time the little-i feels threatened the instinctive survival mechanisms of fight, flight, or freeze get triggered in your autonomic nervous system. These responses have their origin in the reptilian brain. The main job of the reptilian brain, which humans share with most animals, is to guarantee physical survival. In any given moment—by the millisecond, in fact—this part of the brain alerts the organism of a perceived threat and fires one of three survival responses.

In the book, *Waking the Tiger*, Peter Levine writes, "For the reptile, conscious choice is not an option. Every behavior, every movement is instinctual."*3 The same is true for the little-i; your survival response evolved along the same lines as reptilian defense mechanisms.

Independent of what stimulated the negative experience—whether an event in the internal or external world—the defense mechanism will be activated all the same. In other words, you will fight, freeze, or flee in response to both internal and external threats. The only difference is that when there is an external stimulus, you will discharge your aggressive energy towards the actual source of the threat in the case of the fight response. For example, you might yell at a restaurant waitress after waiting half an hour for your food. The same applies for the flight response. If the negative experience is associated with an

external stimulus, you will run away or withdraw from the exterior disturbance, for example the nagging family member, the moody colleague, or the
high-pitched noise of a braking train.

If the fight response of the little-i is directed against yourself, then you will
become aggressive and attack yourself with self-rejection, self-criticism, or self-
blame. As I mentioned before, nothing is more hurtful, causes greater pain,
and forms a larger chasm between you and your natural state of being over
the course of your lifetime than your ongoing self-attack and self-denigration.

The second survival response, flight, means that the little-i is trying to
avoid a negative experience by withdrawing attention from it and repressing
its content. As we discussed in Chapter 3, nothing that you reject will ever
fully disappear. All these criticized, attacked, rejected, and repressed experiences remain hidden in the subconscious realm of your bodymind. Locked
away from your conscious awareness, they become part of the shadow layer.

The shock response, the third survival mechanism, occurs when your
organism is completely overwhelmed in the face of a terrifying experience.
The organism cannot defend itself against the source of the threat by either
attacking it or running away, so the nervous system goes into a state of overwhelm which causes the bodymind to *freeze*. Characterized by dissociation and
numbness, the shock response is often provoked by some crisis, for example:
a tragic accident that results in the loss of a limb, the suicide of a loved one,
or physical violence. Shock is the inability of the bodymind to deal with a
life threatening experience in a self-empowering way and to protect itself effi-
ciently against the source of the threat and its damaging impact.

THE little-i CAN NEVER BE HAPPY

You can imagine the 4 Basic Wants as four hungry and gaping mouths—
the insatiable appetites of the little-i. Each mouth represents one of the 4
Basic Wants. No matter how much food the little-i tries to feed them, the four
mouths will never be satisfied. None of these four mouths can ever get enough:
the *safety-hungry-mouth* never feels safe enough, the *control-hungry-mouth* can
never get enough control, the *love-hungry-mouth* never feels appreciated and
loved enough, and the *satisfaction-hungry-mouth* simply cannot get its fill, and
therefore screams along with Mick Jagger, "I can't get no satisfaction."

Occasionally the four mouths are fed with such *exquisite food*, such an outstanding content of experience, that their appetites temporarily quiet down; for example you have a truly mind-blowing orgasm, get the good news of having passed the final exam after many years of studying, or find out that the person you are in love with loves you, too. What happens in these auspicious instances? The content of experience is of such a majestic quality that the four mouths literally shut up in order to savor this stupendous bite. In this rare moment your mind becomes still and you become aware of your inner Self, your Inner Sun that permeates you with love and happiness.

Attempting to make your little-i enduringly happy is futile, however, since its four hungry mouths suffer from the incurable condition of constant lack. The 4 Basic Wants can never be satisfied regardless of how many good experiences the hungry mouths devour. Extraordinary incidents where you feel truly happy have nothing to do with your little-i. On the contrary, it is the absence of the reactive behavior of the little-i when it momentarily shuts up that allows the warming rays of your Inner Sun to shine into your conscious awareness.

Always too soon however, the happiness fades away as the little-i resur-faces. Once its four mouths have chewed up the ecstatic bite, the next hunger wave emerges and with it the 4 Basic Wants and the reactive behavior pattern of the little-i. And the chase after good experiences, after new food for its four hungry mouths, starts anew. Your *survival gang*—the mask, the inner critic, and the little-i—form an intimate threesome that I like to call *the gang*. Together the three gang members share one basic intention: to secure the survival of the sense of "i". Each member, as I have shared with you, has its own unique strategy for achieving this end.

The world of your survival gang revolves exclusively around the preservation and gratification of their possessive stance toward all things associated with *I-me-mine*. When the mask, the inner critic, or the little-i say, "I", they truly mean the vulnerable, reactive "i" that is the very center of their existence. They all defend and protect you from negative and potentially life-threatening experiences—at least they try to and believe it to be their job. For reasons of simplicity you can imagine the little-i as the boss of the gang, the head of this egocentric threesome, while the mask and the inner critic make up the body of the gang. The mask and the inner critic do whatever they can to guarantee the survival of the gang leader who is the center of their egocentric existence.

THE REACTION PATTERN OF THE little-i

**Whenever you are *lost* in your experience you behave
in a *reactive manner*.**

The following diagram graphically summarizes the previous information of this chapter and shows how the unconscious mechanisms play out when you become completely identified with your here and now experience and as a result react from your little-i—either in an enamored and attached or an averse and resistant manner. This structured illustration further demonstrates how the little-i evaluates the content of your experience and how any opposition to a basic want automatically triggers the survival responses of the reptilian brain.

The Reaction Pattern of the "little-i"

Identification with Your Experience
The little-i is completely
identified with the experience

**Automatic – Unconscious Evaluation
of the Content of Your Experience
based on the 4 Basic Wants:**
- the want to feel / be safe
- the want to feel / be satisfied
- the want to feel / be loved
- the want to feel / be in control

"Good / Positive Experience"
(= desirable / pleasurable)
fulfills one or more of
the 4 Basic Wants

"Bad / Negative Experience"
(= uncomfortable / scary / painful)
does <u>not</u> fulfill any of
the 4 Basic Wants

Evokes Attraction & Attachment
= going for the experience –
wanting it & indulging in it

Triggers Resistance / Aversion /
and / or **Survival Response**

Fight

**Attacking / Aggressing /
Going against**
- (Self-) Rejection
- (Self-) Criticism
- (Self-) Blaming
- Imposition of one's
  will against resistance

Flight

**Going Away From /
Avoiding /
Withdrawing**
- Running away
- Repression

Freeze

**Feeling
Overwhelmed –
Going into Shock /
Paralysis**
- Numbness
- Dissociation
- "Blanking out"

The *Big Eye*—your inner observer

Loving yourself requires becoming aware of your here & now experience.

The inner observer is never lost in your experience because it never becomes identified with content. It simply notices your experience and remains unaffected. Remember that you may choose to exercise the option of going into witness mode at any point during the reaction pattern of the little-i. In other words: in any situation, you can make a conscious choice to step out of your reaction (even if you are in the middle of it), center yourself, and observe your here and now experience in a neutral and detached way from the position of the inner observer. Every time you intentionally *re-center yourself in the inner observer*, you build and strengthen self-awareness.

You are the sole owner of your experience_

Your experience is always your experience & you are responsible for what you do with it.

Your experience is your experience. It does not matter who or what triggers your experience, or what the actual content of your experience is. It does not even matter if you like the content of your experience or not. It is always your experience. You are always the sole owner of your experience.

As human beings we have a tendency to make other people or outer circumstances responsible for our so-called negative experiences. If you observe yourself closely you might catch yourself blaming your partner, a family member, your neighbor, your boss, a colleague, the economy, the weather, human nature, life, or God for your current unhappiness. When you are in a blaming mood you make statements such as:

"You make me feel…"
"Because of you I feel…"
"Its your fault that I feel…"
"You are the one who…"

"If only you were different (not like...) then I could be happy."

You can complete each sentence in your own way while thinking of the person or situation you tend to blame for your negative experiences. Whenever you blame another person you make her/him responsible for your experience and, in so doing, give up your sovereignty and personal power. If you try to disown your experience by blaming yourself, by judging yourself, and by making yourself wrong for having a negative experience, you compound the injury and hurt yourself even more. For example, say you fail an exam or lose money in the stock market and start berating yourself with thoughts such as: *I'm such a loser, what an idiot I turned out to be...* In addition to the pain you feel at having lost something of value, you add the pain of self-attack. In other words, you push yet another ping pong ball down into your shadow layer by disowning and repressing the unwanted aspects of your experience. Relatively unaware, you have just increased the separation between you and your Inner Sun and cut yourself off from the source of love and happiness within you.

The truth is you are the owner of your experience and therefore you are responsible for what you do with the content of your experience. If you blame or attack someone for an experience that you are currently having, then this is your choice of how to deal with it. The other person might accept your blame and truly believe that s/he is responsible for your negative experience; likewise, that is her/his choice. But regardless of who you blame for your experience, and how much that person goes along with the blame-dance, you are still its owner and you always will be. Thus, it is up to you how you relate to your experience and what you subsequently do with it.

You are not your experience—only its "temporary owner".

If you've got a dog and he kills a few chickens on your neighbor's farm, it is your responsibility and you will be expected to pay the damages. You are not your dog, however, because you are his owner you are responsible for what he does. The same is true for your experience. You are not your experience—you are much more than that—but you are its owner and, therefore, responsible for what you do with it.

Making others or outer life circumstances responsible for your experience is a common human practice, especially when you are confronted with uncomfortable, scary, or painful contents. In reality, your attempt to disown your experience—to get rid of it, reject it, repress it, or blame others for it—is a hopeless effort. You may not like what you are experiencing, and you may wish you could make it go away by handing it off to someone else, but this will never work. All of your experiences belong to you just as your body belongs to you. Disowning an experience is like disowning a part of your body. Next time you find yourself blaming someone for an experience that you are having, you can imagine that what you are really trying to do is to get rid of some part of your body—for example your arm, foot, or hand—by making her/him the new owner of it. Obviously we cannot make someone else the owner of a part of our body or a certain experience, and yet this is exactly what we humans do when we blame others for experiences we don't like.

You live in your bodymind with all its experiences & it is your choice how you respond to it.

If you don't own your here and now experience—if you don't take responsibility for it—you are at the mercy of the unconscious reaction pattern of the little-i. Living reactively, making others responsible for your negative experiences, is a form of self-victimization. This tendency keeps you powerless since you abandon your capacity to consciously choose how you will relate to yourself and the content of your experience.

There is nothing, no experience that you can ever discard or disown. As stated in Chapter 3, repressed experiences *go underground* and become part of your shadow self. The more you repress, the thicker this shadow layer grows and the harder it is for you to consciously access your Inner Sun, the source of love and happiness within you.

INNER & OUTER ATTITUDE

"It's not what happens to you,
but how you respond to it that matters."
Epictetus

Your *inner attitude* is your inner posture, or *feeling mindset*, that determines how you relate to your here and now experience. As you have read in the previous chapter, the only thing you ever have and ever can relate to is your own experience. Therefore your inner attitude is always directed towards your inner experience, independent of whether its content is triggered by a stimulus of your internal (a memory, for example) or external world (such as a friend).

Your inner attitude is constantly mirrored in your body posture and your outer attitude of how you relate to the external world.

Your inner attitude is how you relate to your inner experience; your outer attitude is how you relate to your environment and your fellow human beings. The emphasis in this book is on your inner attitude—how you relate to your experience within yourself. Whenever I use the word *attitude* from here on, I will be referring to this inner attitude whether I explicitly say so or not. You always have an attitude towards yourself—an attitude of how you relate to your here and now experience. The quality of your inner attitude is always reflected in your outer attitude: in your body posture, your movements, your gestures, your facial expressions, the way you breathe, and the sound of your voice. Even if you don't say a word, another person intuitively reads your body language and thus gets a *feeling-impression* of your general state of being and your attitude towards her/him. Your body posture is the mirror of your inner attitude.

If you feel open and relaxed, at ease with yourself, then your physical body will show it in an open, receptive, and inviting body posture. You will breathe from your belly in a slow and even manner. Your eyes will move about slowly and look at everything with a mellow quality. Your facial expression will express an inner contentment, and your overall movements will be smooth and graceful. If, on the other hand, you feel anxious, nervous, and restless, you will breathe from your chest in a rather quick and shallow fashion. Your body movements will be quick, hurried, and uncoordinated. You might find yourself performing some unintentional, repetitive movements like tapping your fingers or moving your foot up and down. Such nervous movements are an attempt to discharge some of this agitated and excessive energy within your bodymind. For example, you may have a tendency to cross your arms or legs when you feel insecure and need protection and containment.

People know instinctively what your inner attitude is in a given moment; your body posture tells them right away whether it is safe to approach and interact with you. One only needs to look at you and read your body signals in order to find out if your attitude is open and friendly, closed and reserved, or hostile and aggressive.

Usually, you are not consciously choosing your inner attitude, but reacting in your old, habitual ways.

You always have an inner attitude towards your experience, but most people don't choose their attitude consciously. Disconnected from the inner observer, and thus unaware of your here and now experience, you find yourself locked up in the cage of the reactive behavior pattern of the little-i. Lost in the content of your experience, you behave like a robot that cannot actively choose its inner attitude and the way it wants to relate to its experiences. The lack of self-awareness turns you into a victim of your own experience and your habitual reaction pattern, as they are described in the diagram of the reaction pattern of the little-i, on page 82 . But the good new is, at any moment in your life, you also have the potential to become aware of your here and now experi-ence and to consciously own it. As you cultivate your self-awareness, the inner observer gives you the freedom to choose your attitude and how you want to respond to your here and now experience. This simple shift empowers you to live a conscious life.

"There is a little difference in people, but that little difference makes a big difference. That little difference is attitude."
W. Clement Stone

YOUR FREEDOM OF CHOICE

"Everything can be taken away from a man but one thing: the
last of the human freedom—to choose one's attitude in any
given set of circumstances, to choose one's own way."
Viktor Frankl,
Austrian Psychiatrist - Survivor of the Holocaust

The Inner
Observer

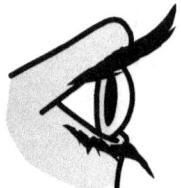

The Content
of Experience

The "Big Eye"
...is aware of...
...is conscious of...
...perceives...

"If you are aware or conscious of your here & now experience,
then you have the freedom to choose your inner attitude—the
"how" with which you relate to the content of your
experience."

"A healthy attitude is contagious but don't wait
to catch it from others. Be a carrier."
Source Unknown

The greatest freedom you possess as a human being is the ability to choose your inner attitude. Your inner attitude is the fundamental factor that determines the quality of your life. Everything shifts—how you relate to your here and now experience, how you experience yourself, your fellow human beings, and your environment—when you choose an inner attitude that is grounded in self-acceptance and Selflove.

> **"What creates our freedom, or our lack,**
> **is our attitude toward whatever we meet."**
> Charlotte Selver

YOU CHOOSE YOUR ATTITUDE

It's always you who chooses your inner attitude,
consciously or unconsciously. Nobody else!

You always have an attitude. In every moment of your life you have an attitude towards everything that you experience. You have no choice about that. You cannot choose not to have an attitude, the same as you cannot choose to no longer take on a certain body posture. Since you always have an attitude, I encourage you to make intentional use of your free will and to decide *how* you want to relate to your experience. Rather than just relying on an unconscious atti-tude towards your experience, purposely choose one that serves you the best.

> **"I believe the single most significant decision I can make on a**
> **day-to-day basis is my choice of attitude."**
> Charles Swindoll

Have you ever considered consciously establishing and cultivating a permanent inner attitude that will accompany you like a best friend and wise teacher throughout your life? Independent of what you are going through, or what your current experience will be, this attitude remains. Is the possibility of developing such a basic attitude attractive to you? - Then let's get started.

CHOOSING TO CULTIVATE A LOVING ATTITUDE TOWARDS YOURSELF

To love yourself means to consciously relate to your here and now experience with a loving attitude.

I invite you now to make the choice to cultivate a loving attitude towards all aspects of yourself, towards all of your experiences, independent of their contents. The cultivation of a loving attitude towards all of your experiences, including your resistance and reaction against the initial experience, is the very foundation of Selflove. This is the way to become your own best friend.

THE 2ND STEP OF THE ART OF SELFLOVE

The Inner Observer

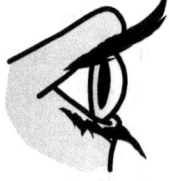

The Content of Experience

The "Big Eye"

...chooses a loving attitude...   ...towards the content of experience.

Meeting your experiences, including your resistance and reactions against your experiences, with a loving attitude represents the 2nd step of the Art of Selflove.

The 2nd step of the Art of Selflove empowers you to meet all of your experiences, even your resistance, your aversions and reactions against the actual content with a loving attitude.

This means it will no longer matter what you experience, whether you are feeling angry, sad, frustrated, afraid, moody, cranky, lonely, upset, depressed, envious, jealous, bored, shy, insecure, embarrassed, distrustful, nervous, impatient, demanding, greedy, worried, aloof, resistant, reluctant, or whatever... you simply relate to your here and now experience, or your reaction against it, with a loving attitude.

> **"Our attitudes control our lives. Attitudes are**
> **a secret power working twenty-four hours a day,**
> **for good or bad. It is of paramount importance that**
> **we know how to harness and control this great force."**
> Tom Blandi

Do you think you can learn to cultivate a loving attitude towards all of your experience, towards all aspects of yourself, to love yourself and to be your own best friend, in every situation of your life, no matter what?

Yes, you can; by cultivating a basic and loving attitude towards all of yourself, towards all of your experiences. How do you do it practically, not just theoretically? How do you apply the Art of Selflove in your daily life? How do you become aware of your here and now experience? How do you cultivate a loving attitude towards all of your experiences, even your reactions against them? This is exactly what the Welcoming-Process is designed to help you accomplish.

In the next section you will learn how to *harness* this great power of a loving attitude.

PART THREE

"The Selflove-Practice"

CHAPTER 6

The Welcoming-Process™ - The Key to Cultivating the Art of Selflove

YOU are about to get your hands on one of the most valuable skills you may ever acquire: the ability to love yourself. The Welcoming-Process crystallizes and synthesizes my lifelong search for a simple, yet powerful way to *live ever more fully in and out of the love that I am—and that we all are— at the core.* Years of intense introspection, self-analysis, contemplation, and experimentation with yoga and personal therapy, as well as pioneering studies in holistic healing and somatic education in the US and Switzerland, went into developing this method. It is the cornerstone of my private practice as a Somatic Therapist and Body-Centered Life Coach. The Art of Selflove begins when you decide to cultivate a conscious and loving relationship with yourself. No amount of money, success, or love will fully satisfy you or bring you lasting happiness if you haven't learned to love yourself. Nothing *out there*, not even the most adoring friend or life partner, can take away the self-mutilating pain of your inner war. The Welcoming-Process is a simple and practical tool that will enable you to begin loving yourself and become your own best friend. And the more you learn to love yourself with all of your experiences, the easier it will be for you to love others with theirs.

WHAT IS THE WELCOMING-PROCESS?

The Welcoming-Process is a powerful & straightforward 3-step method to cultivate the Art of Selflove; the skill to love yourself and to become your own best friend.

Everybody interested in learning the Welcoming-Process can do so easily with the help of this book. All you need to do is learn and practice three simple and clearly structured steps, which are outlined in detail in the coming chapters and summarized—in a simplified manner—in the diagram of the Welcoming-Cycle™ on page 147.

The Welcoming-Process is:

- **A simple & powerful 3-step method to cultivate the Art of Selflove**
- **A mindfulness practice to reinforce the inner observer**
- **A way to relate consciously**
- **A way to develop a loving attitude towards yourself & all of your experiences**
- **A way of loving yourself & others**
- **A way to live harmoniously**
- **A way to befriend yourself & to become your own best friend**

BENEFITS OF THE WELCOMING-PROCESS

What can you expect to get from practicing the Welcoming-Process?

Practicing the Welcoming-Process on a regular basis will help you:

- Transform & harmonize your negative self-talk, self-attack, and bad moods
- Develop a consistent, loving attitude towards yourself and all your experiences

- Increase your self-esteem, self-worth, and self-confidence
- Cultivate your inner observer for greater self-awareness & mindfulness
- Learn to relate to all of your experiences in a conscious & loving way, including the uncomfortable ones
- Empower yourself by taking responsibility for your experiences
- Become ever more grounded in your body
- Connect with your Inner Self—the source of love & happiness
- Feel more loved, happy, and whole *from within*
- Rely confidently on your inner authority
- Feel calmer, more balanced, and more centered in the here & now
- Expand your inner sense of freedom
- Deepen your attentiveness of your inner voice
- Gain greater understanding & compassion for yourself & others
- Consciously choose what, how, when, and to whom you express yourself
- Create more harmonious relationships
- Master the art of loving yourself & others

I know the same way I and others continue to enjoy all of the above benefits, so can you as you learn the Welcoming-Process and begin to use it regularly in your own life.

An imaginary story to illustrate what the Welcoming-Process "does"

Imagine you live in a heavily polluted industrial mega city where you never see the sun. Factories and motor vehicles spew toxic fumes into the atmosphere day and night; the sky above looks blackish-grey. Having lived in this city all your life it would be easy to believe, as some people do, that the sun is just a legend. But you remember a day long ago when a gale force wind ripped a hole in the clouds and gave you a glimpse of a gorgeous blue sky. You will never forget the intense joy that filled your whole being when you saw the sun and felt those warm rays caress your face. The memory of that dazzling round has never left you. Touched by a sublime and other-worldly dimension, you know deep inside that true happiness exists. You and everyone you know

have given up wallpaper and once-popular faux-painted walls in favor of the latest in home-décor: ultra-thin cinema displays that cover the walls and ceilings. Projected onto these screens is an ever changing, 24-hour virtual weather pattern. Rather than getting up to see the sunrise on the horizon, you see it rise on your nature-screens. When you come home from a hard days work, you watch a virtual sunset splash its spectacular colors across mountains, lakes, or rolling hills, depending on what landscape you have programmed. The position of the sun, as well as the length of each day, changes with the seasons. At night you see a vast night sky filled with stars projected onto your ceiling-mounted nature-screens. The constellations disappear gradually as night gives way to the dawn of a new day, just as they would out in nature.

Referring to Reich's model of the 3 Layered Self that we looked at in Chapter 3, the rarely glimpsed sun is your real Self at the core level, which is depicted as the primary layer. The second layer, or shadow self, is the polluted atmosphere—the dark, blackish-gray sky. Your apartment with its 24-hour virtual weather pattern is the third layer, your mask and ideal self. In the *ideal world* of your apartment you are no longer confronted with the pain and suffering that comes with living a nature-deprived existence without clean air, sunshine, birds, trees, and blue skies. Your nature-screens give you a sense of comfort and wellbeing by helping you ignore the gloomy and hostile world you live in.

Symbolically speaking, the Welcoming-Process is a powerful, human-friendly technology that has the potential to transform this industrial mega city with its apocalyptic sky back into an authentically beautiful natural environment. The process is applied in a step-by-step manner: one issue, one topic, one experience; one smoking chimney, one factory, one car exhaust, and one heating system at a time. There is no rush, no panic, just steady progress. Every factory that starts to implement the new *Welcoming-technology* immediately starts to produce energy in an environmentally friendly way. This frees up additional energy and resources which can then be put to use purifying the remaining contaminates in the atmosphere. Each time you use the Welcoming-Process to deal with an issue in your life, another factory, another home, another car in your mega-city is transformed and harmonized. The more you use this process in your life, the more you *clean up* your shadow layer. Over time the wall screens in your apartment that display an ideal, virtual sky lose their allure. You become much more in touch with and fascinated by the real sky that is now clearing up and becoming less gloomy. Your shadow patches give way to an inner sense of lightness and happiness. The rays of your Inner Sun and your essential qualities can shine through the dark atmosphere more often. In such moments you realize, "Wow, the Inner Sun, the source of love and happiness really exists! It is inside of me and it is who I truly am."

I don't know how long it takes to purify all of the dark clouds and shadow patches. My inner atmosphere still needs a lot of Selflove since there are still more unattended and toxic factories polluting my inner world. At the same time, each time I am able to transform and harmonize another issue, another theme, another "smoking chimney" with the assistance of the Welcoming-Process, the immediate relief in the way I feel encourages me to keep going, one step at a time. Each bit of effort is clearly another step in the right direction towards more light, love, and happiness.

THE WELCOMING-PROCESS IS A "WRITTEN PROCESS"

In general the Welcoming-Process is a *written process*. Especially in the beginning while you are still becoming familiar with it, it is important that you write down each of the 3 steps. In Chapter 11, I will explain how you can take yourself through the written part of the process in a very fast and efficient way. I highly recommend that you get a journal, a personal *Selflove-Journal* to keep track of your *Welcoming-Sessions*, as well as any thoughts, ideas, issues, or questions that come up while reading this book. Get in the habit of having your Selflove-Journal close at hand so that you can use it wherever you are—at home in bed, on the subway, in the office, at a restaurant, on a park bench, out in nature, or wherever.

Your Selflove-Journal is like a faithful companion that supports you in practicing the Art of Selflove in your daily life and thus in becoming your own best friend.

INVITATION TO PERSONALIZE YOUR SELFLOVE-JOURNAL

The following steps are an invitation to give your Selflove-Journal a personal touch. If you are not interested in personalizing your Selflove-Journal, you can skip this section and go straight to the next heading, *The power of writing*.

1. Buy your Selflove-Journal and a pen you enjoy writing with.
2. Go to a place where you feel at ease & make yourself comfortable.
3. Choose one of the following terms or sentences you feel most drawn to:

   - Selflove
   - Loving Myself
   - "I am my own best friend."
   - "I love myself."

4. Close your eyes and take a few deep breaths into your belly. Feel how your belly expands as you inhale and how it flattens as you exhale. Enjoy the deepening of relaxation.
5. Silently keep repeating the term of your choice with a feeling of love and observe the image, symbol, thought, sentence, word, or association that comes to your mind.
6. When something has come to mind, open your eyes, turn to the first page of your Selflove-Journal, and create your own personal front page using this image, symbol, or word. For example, you might get the image of a sun, a flower, or a rainbow. If you like to you can give your journal your own name or title as well.

Having personalized your Selflove-Journal you are ready to start using it for the upcoming exercises and eventually for your own Welcoming-Sessions.

The power of writing

Writing supports the inner observer in you and strengthens your ability to contain yourself with the content of your experience.

Writing is a very powerful process or technique in itself, one that numerous spiritual paths use as a vital form of meditation. According to the American Psychology Association*1, the positive effect of writing is supported by empirical evidence: "...writing is an easy, inexpensive, independent and relatively universal way for people [to] resist the mental and physical ravages of stress and disease." Furthermore: "Anyone who has benefited from keeping a diary or a journal can further justify the time and effort, secure in the knowledge that disclosing innermost thoughts and feelings—even or especially about bad experiences—is good for health." Given the fact that I have been journaling since I was eighteen, I can fully confirm the findings of these studies based on my own writing practice; primarily the ease and speed with which you can move through intensely stressful situations and the clarity you gain from writing about your experience.

Writing is truly a highly effective means of developing and cultivating the inner observer. As you write your experience into your journal you automatically *take a step back*, which allows you to put some distance between yourself and the actual content of your experience. In other words, it enables us to become objective about what is usually subjective. Writing also helps you build up your self-containment; the ability to contain the content of your experience, basically all that you sense, feel, think, desire, and imagine inside. The more you can contain yourself, the less likely you are to lose control and *act out* in an unconscious and reactive manner, as I described in the reaction pattern of the little-i, on page 82. This *inner container* places you in a position to make a conscious choice: if you want to share and express your inner experience with a friend, for example. And if so, to decide how, when, and what part of your experience you will share. The writing component of the Welcoming-Process is not only a training tool to become more familiar with the actual process but it also empowers you to make conscious use of your human birthright and privilege: your freedom to choose how you want to relate to yourself and others.

THE EXCEPTION: WHEN YOU GET "TRIGGERED ON THE SPOT"

The consistent practice of writing down your Welcoming-Sessions gives you the solid foundation to do the Welcoming-Process spontaneously, *just in your mind.*

Writing down your Welcoming-Session is the best preparation and training for you to be able to use the Welcoming-Process spontaneously when your *buttons get pushed,* which is to say when you are suddenly caught up in a reactive pattern. Every time you are in the middle of an emotionally upsetting situation, you do the Welcoming-Process right on the spot. Say for example, your partner offends you by being cranky, or your boss is harsh in how he criticizes your work. Straightaway, you can do the Welcoming-Process in your head, without stopping to write it down. Once you have practiced the process often enough that it becomes second nature to you, you can use it in the heat of daily living, especially when you get triggered and need your own loving the most. To be able to love yourself while in the midst of problematic situations is not a superfluous luxury but an indispensable necessity, and that is why it is so important that you write down your Welcoming-Sessions consistently.

THE 3 BASIC STEPS OF THE WELCOMING-PROCESS

The 3 steps of the Welcoming-Process:

1st **Step - Welcoming**
2nd **Step - Allowing**
3rd **Step - Noticing-the-Bodyshift**

The 3 steps of the Welcoming-Process are the distilled, practical essence of all the theoretical information of the previous chapters on *How to Cultivate the Art of Selflove.*

I will guide you systematically, step-by-step, through the Welcoming-Process. In each of the next three chapters I will present one step of the process, which will make it very easy to become familiar with each of the three steps. The information is very detailed and extensive to make sure that you get a thorough understanding of each of the three steps. You don't need to actively remember all this information. What matters is that you fully understand the main points in the framed textboxes and that you do the exercises as you go along. Remember you are learning a new skill, so please be patient with yourself and enjoy the ride!

CHAPTER 7

"WELCOMING" - The 1st Step of the Welcoming-Process

"The Truth will set you free."
John 8:31-32

A S you know, the first step in the Art of Selflove is to become aware of your here and now experience, your subjective truth in the present moment. *Welcoming,* the 1ˢᵗ Step of the Welcoming-Process, is a conscious choice to make contact with your experience and to recognize its content exactly as it is. When you *welcome* your experience, you intentionally relate to whatever is happening by honestly acknowledging that which you sense, need, feel, think, or imagine.

Metaphorically speaking, *Welcoming* is like turning on a flashlight in a dark room so that you can see what you were previously unaware of. Just because you cannot see a tree in the dark does not mean that it is not there. The same is true for the various contents of your experience; certain feelings, dreams, desires, or thoughts from the past or the present tend to go unnoticed unless you choose to welcome them into your awareness. Just because you are not aware of them does not mean that they are not there. They might just be invisible to you, hidden in the darkness of your subconscious. *Welcoming* shines the light of awareness onto the tree (the content of your experience) so that you can become fully aware of its existence, and fully recognize it as it is, including its size and location.

> **"Welcoming" means you consciously choose to contact your here & now experience and become familiar with its content as it is.**

The journey of loving yourself starts where you are right now; with *Welcoming* your here & now experience.

HOW DO YOU ACCOMPLISH "WELCOMING"?

I.
Ask yourself <u>one</u>*
of
the "Welcoming-Questions":

"What are you experiencing right now?"
"What is your experience right now?"
"What is your here & now experience?"

"What do you notice right now?"
"What do you perceive right now?"
"What do you observe right now?"

The *Welcoming-Question*
assists you in becoming aware of
the content of your here & now experience.

2.
Write Down Your Answer!
= the content of your here & now experience

*Choose the Welcoming-Question you like best, since any of them will directly bring you into contact with the content of your here & now experience.

The simple formula for the "Welcoming-Step"

1.	**Ask <u>One</u>* of the Welcoming-Questions** For example: "What are you experiencing right now?"
2.	**Write Down Your Answer - that's it!**

---

*For the purpose of variety and your own preference you can choose from a selection of different Welcoming-Questions. If you decide not to make use of the various Welcoming-Questions, but prefer to always ask the same question, this is a totally valid choice as well.

When have you completed the Welcoming-Step?

**When you have written down your answer
– the actual content of your here & now experience -
you have completed the Welcoming-Step.
Then you are ready to go on to the 2nd Step of the
Welcoming-Process.**

---

10 Practical examples of "Welcoming"

What follows is a list of ten examples of the Welcoming-Step, taken from various Welcoming-Sessions. These are offered to familiarize you with the process, to demonstrate the use of the various welcoming questions, and to show a range of experiential contents that can be welcomed in this way.

1) **1st Step - Welcoming: What are you experiencing right now?**
   "There is some tightness in my left shoulder."
2) **1st Step - Welcoming: What is your experience right now?**
   "I feel a mixture of excitement and anxiety."

3) **1ˢᵗ Step - Welcoming: What is your here & now experience?**
"I fear that I might be criticized when I do nothing and just relax."

4) **1ˢᵗ Step - Welcoming: What do you notice right now?**
"It is my dream to live in my own house."

5) **1ˢᵗ Step - Welcoming: What is your here & now experience?**
"I keep running away from my fears and worries."

6) **1ˢᵗ Step - Welcoming: What do you perceive right now?**
"I feel scared of what will happen when I say "no" to my partner."

7) **1ˢᵗ Step - Welcoming: What are you experiencing right now?**
"I shouldn't think so negatively."

8) **1ˢᵗ Step - Welcoming: What do you observe right now?**
"I want to earn more money."

9) **1ˢᵗ Step - Welcoming: What are you experiencing right now?**
"I am resistant to getting in touch with my sadness."

10) **1ˢᵗ Step - Welcoming: What is your here & now experience?**
"Why haven't I laughed in such a long time?"*

* Sometimes the content of your experience comes in the form of a question as well.

THE ONLY-ONE-CONTENT RULE OF THE WELCOMING-STEP

"Little by little does the trick."
Aesop (620-560 BC)

**"WELCOME" only one content of experience
in one Welcoming-Step**

The main reason for the *only-one-content rule* is to make sure that you do not overwhelm yourself when you deal with challenging or highly charged emotional issues, such as relational conflicts, health problems, or financial worries. By addressing only one content in each Welcoming-Step you *break down* the overall issue or theme into more easy-to-digest portions of experience; this allows the process to proceed organically, as you will soon see. And while life may seem to come at you in massive oceanic waves, this practice reveals the remarkable ability of your awareness to swallow that ocean one thimbleful at a time.

The practice of choosing only one content of experience in one Welcoming-Step requires some discipline in the beginning. But you will soon realize that doing so is what makes the Welcoming-Process such a safe and powerful method. This is especially true when you are dealing with a *hot potato*—a difficult problem or demanding issue that brings up intense discomfort or strong emotions such as worry, fear, frustration, rage, jealousy, grief, etc.

EXERCISE TO BECOME FAMILIAR WITH THE WELCOMING-STEP

"A journey of a 1000 miles starts with a first step."
Lao-Tse

You are about to take your first step in practicing the Welcoming-Process. Mastering the Art of Selflove is truly a lifelong journey, for all aspects of you and all of your experiences long to be loved, consciously recognized, and *welcomed* just as they are.

Since this exercise is just a preparation to become familiar with the Welcoming-Process, it is important to be in a relaxed, comfortable, and somewhat neutral or positive state when you do it. In other words, don't pick a hot potato to experiment with just yet. Once you are familiar with the process, you can readily take yourself through it when you feel emotionally upset or uneasy inside. But if you are really agitated and upset it is not the right moment to do this initial exercise. Wait until you feel more at ease again.

PRACTICING THE WELCOMING-STEP

1. Write in your Selflove-Journal the heading, *Practicing the Welcoming-Step*
2. Choose <u>one</u> of the Welcoming-Questions and write it down.
3. Mentally ask yourself the Welcoming-Question.
4. Write down your answer (= the content of your experience) Example:
   1ˢᵗ Step: "Welcoming" - What are you experiencing right now? - "I feel frustrated."

5. Keep repeating points 2 through 4 until you have *welcomed* ten contents of experience. Number each Welcoming-Step sequence from 1 -10. You can always choose the same Welcoming-Question or a different one depending on what you prefer.

The practical examples of the Welcoming-Steps on pages 107 & 108 give you an exact visual outline of how to do this exercise. As I mentioned before, I will show you the short version of writing down each of the 3 Steps of the Welcoming-Process later in this book (see page 170). For now it is useful to write down the Welcoming-Question every time because this will allow you to become thoroughly familiar with the Welcoming-Step.

"WELCOMING" IS A PATH OF CULTIVATING
THE INNER OBSERVER

A client called me a few days after being introduced to the Welcoming-Process and said, "It is quite amazing! The inner observer is present all the time. Since I left your place, after you explained it to me, I constantly notice how I observe myself. I have not even begun yet with the other two steps of the process. When I left, I was a bit skeptical about your method because it seemed too simple for it to work. But the Welcoming-Step really cultivates the inner observer!"

I was very happy to get his feedback, because becoming aware of the inner observer is the exact intention behind the Welcoming-Step. As you know from the previous chapters, first you need to become aware of yourself—of your *inner world*, your bodymind, your here and now experience—before you are able to choose to relate to it with a loving attitude. The Welcoming-Step trains you to grow ever more conscious of the inner observer; this is the prerequisite to cultivating the Art of Selflove.

Many meditation practices, especially those that come from Eastern traditions, focus exclusively on the process of self-observation in order to develop *mindfulness,* which automatically strengthens awareness of the inner observer in the practitioner. In Eastern traditions such as Taoism, a spiritual path is also called a *path of inner cultivation*. Any such path requires a regular prac-tice to establish the inner observer. This is exactly what the Welcoming-Step, the 1st step of the Welcoming-Process, will do for you as you use it regularly.

Every time you apply the Welcoming-Step, you practice the art of mindfulness and expand your ability to simply be aware of your here and now experience.

"Mindfulness is honest introspection, helping us see things as they actually are."
Tara Bennet-Goleman

CHAPTER 8

"ALLOWING" - The 2nd Step of the Welcoming-Process

**"Pain exists only in resistance
Joy exists only in acceptance
Painful situations which you heartily accept become joyful
Joyful situations which you do not accept become painful
There is no such thing as a bad experience
Bad experiences are simply the creations of
your resistance to what is."**
Rumi

ALLOWING is the 2nd Step of the Welcoming-Process. This practical key opens the door to a loving attitude towards all of your experiences, including all your reactions, aversions, and resistances. *Allowing* and *accepting* are so closely related in their meaning that they are almost interchangeable terms, but not quite. I have chosen the term *Allowing* because it is all-encompassing and even gives a green light to your *non-acceptance*, your *resistance*, your *aversion*, and the "No, not that!" position you take toward the content of your experience. As we dive into this chapter and start practicing the Allowing-Step you will have a firsthand experience of the broader and more transformative effect of allowing when compared to acceptance. In my experience, acceptance often comes with a dash of forcefulness or resignation, whereas allowing has no such connotation or flavor. Practice the method and decide for yourself. What we are aiming for here is a total embrace of your here and now experience.

Allowing is the all-loving, all-embracing attitude towards all of
your experiences, independent of what the actual content is.
Allowing even embraces your non-acceptance, your dislike, and
your resistance against your here & now experience.

"Life has no other discipline to impose, if we would
but realize it, than to accept life unquestioningly.
Everything we shut our eyes to, everything we run away
from, everything we deny, denigrate or despise,
serves to defeat us in the end.
What seems nasty, painful, evil, can become a source of beauty,
joy and strength, if faced with an open mind. "
Henry Miller

Nathaniel Brandon, the American psychologist who pioneered the field of
self-esteem, said it most succinctly: "The first step toward change is awareness.
The second step is acceptance."*3 Brandon expresses a grand experiential truth
that I intentionally integrated in the first two steps of the Welcoming-Process.

The first step of transformation is *Welcoming.*
The second step is *Allowing.*

Now let's turn our attention to exactly how you practice "allowing" your
experience so that you can verify this for yourself.

How do you accomplish "Allowing"?

1.
Ask Yourself
the "Allowing-Question":

"Can you allow your here & now experience*?"

* The body-sensation, need, feeling, emotion, thought etc...whatever
the content of your experience is, that you have just *Welcomed* & Written
Down in the 1st Step of the Welcoming-Process

2.
Answer the *Allowing-Question* with "Yes" or "No"

Depending on what your truth is:
"Yes!" means: You can allow your experience as it is.
"No!" means: You <u>cannot</u> allow your experience as it is.

3.
Write Down Your Process!
(= the *Allowing-Question* & your answer)

---

10 Practical examples of "Allowing"

Here are a number of examples taken from different Welcoming-Sessions.
These are offered to assist you in clarifying how to apply the Allowing-Step:

1. 1st Step - Welcoming: "I sense restlessness in my body."
    **2nd Step - Allowing: Can you allow sensing restlessness in your
    body? Yes.**
2. 1st Step - Welcoming: "I feel nervous energy."
    2nd Step - Allowing: Can you allow feeling nervous energy? Yes.
3. 1st Step - Welcoming: "I would like to quit my job."
    **2nd Step - Allowing: Can you allow the thought that you would
    like to quit your job? Yes.**

4. 1ˢᵗ Step - Welcoming: "Now my mind is very calm."
    2ⁿᵈ Step - Allowing: Can you allow that your mind is very calm now? Yes.

5. 1ˢᵗ Step - Welcoming: "I remember how afraid I was in this moment."
    2ⁿᵈ Step - Allowing: Can you allow remembering how afraid you were in this moment? Yes.

6. 1ˢᵗ Step - Welcoming: "I feel angry that I'm confronted with this difficult situation."
    2ⁿᵈ Step - Allowing: Can you allow feeling angry that you are confronted with this difficult situation? Yes.

7. 1ˢᵗ Step - Welcoming: "I feel I need more sleep."
    2ⁿᵈ Step - Allowing: Can you allow feeling that you need more sleep? Yes.

8. 1ˢᵗ Step - Welcoming: "I want to have more control in my life."
    2ⁿᵈ Step - Allowing: Can you allow wanting to have more control in your life? Yes.

9. 1ˢᵗ Step - Welcoming: "I just want to lie in bed and do nothing."
    2ⁿᵈ Step - Allowing: Can you allow wanting to lie in bed and do nothing? Yes.

10. 1ˢᵗ Step - Welcoming: "I feel like a failure."
    2ⁿᵈ Step - Allowing: Can you allow feeling like a failure? Yes.

Maybe you have noticed that each of the above *Allowing-Questions* was answered with *Yes*. But what happens if you say, *No*, if you <u>*cannot allow*</u> your here & now experience?

THE "NOT-ALLOWING" OF YOUR EXPERIENCE

On occasion, and at times quite frequently, when you ask the Allowing-Question you will get a clear "No!" This is to be expected; all of us reject our experience at times. But rather than go into denial, distract yourself, or hide from what you are experiencing in some other way, this practice shows you what to do when your response to the Allowing-Question is: "*No*, I cannot allow my experience!" There are three distinct questions, the *3 Not-Allowing-Questions* you can ask yourself when this is the case. Each addresses a slightly different nuance to the *No*.

WHAT DO YOU DO WHEN YOU SAY "NO" TO ALLOWING YOUR EXPERIENCE?

If you say: "No!"
You are saying:
"No, I cannot allow the content of my experience."

Ask yourself <u>one</u>*
of
the "3 Not-Allowing-Questions":

"Can you allow your "No"?"
"Can you allow your "Not-Allowing"?"
"Can you allow your "Resistance"?"

*All three of these <u>*Not-Allowing-Questions*</u> are <u>equally valid</u>.
Choose the one you like the best.

A practical example of how to apply the "3 Not-Allowing-Questions"

1st Step - Welcoming: "I feel very tired."

2nd Step - Allowing: Can you allow this tiredness? *"No!"*

Your "No" is basically saying: "I *cannot allow what is happening*", or "I cannot allow my experience as it is." Every time you say "No" to your experience, the next step is to ask yourself one (only one!) of the *3 Not-Allowing-Questions* in order to continue with the Allowing-Step:

The 3 "Not-Allowing-Questions" are:

1. **"Allowing" the "No":**
   Can you allow your *No*? Yes.
2. **"Allowing" the "Not-Allowing":**
   Can you allow your *Not-Allowing*? Yes.
3. **"Allowing" the "Resistance":**
   Can you allow your *Resistance*? Yes.

Once you have said "Yes" to the Not-Allowing-Question of your choice & written down your answer, you have completed the Allowing-Step.

BASIC RULE IF YOU SAY "NO" TO ALLOWING YOUR EXPERIENCE

Any time you say, "No", and thus cannot allow your here & now experience, continue the Welcoming-Process by asking one* of the 3 Not-Allowing-Questions.

---

* For the purpose of variety and preference you can choose from 3 different Not-Allowing-Questions. If you make the decision to use only one of the 3 questions consistently from here on, this is okay, too.

MORE PRACTICAL EXAMPLES OF NOT-ALLOWING THE CONTENT OF YOUR EXPERIENCE:

1. 1st Step - Welcoming: "I don't feel professionally successful."
   2nd Step - Allowing: Can you allow not feeling professionally successful? **No!**
   Ask One of the Not-Allowing-Questions: **Can you allow your "No"?** Yes

2. 1st Step - Welcoming: "I have no partner, no lover in my life."
   2nd Step - Allowing: Can you allow the experience of not having a partner in your life? **No!**
   Ask One of the Not-Allowing-Questions: **Can you allow your "Not-Allowing"?** Yes.

3. 1st Step - Welcoming: "I don't feel attractive."
   2nd Step - Allowing: Can you allow not feeling attractive? **No!**
   Ask One of the "Not-Allowing-Questions": **Can you allow your "Resistance"?** Yes.

WHAT DO YOU DO IF YOU SAY "NO" TO YOUR NOT-ALLOWING-QUESTION?

"If you _cannot allow_ your "No"*
then simply go back to the 1st Step of the Welcoming-Process
and ask yourself the Welcoming-Question again:

"What are you experiencing right now?"

---

* ("Not-Allowing" or "Resistance")

Example of "Not-Allowing" your "No", "Not-Allowing", or "Resistance":

1st Step - Welcoming: "I lost a lot of money with a bad investment."
2nd Step - Allowing: Can you allow the experience of having lost a lot of money?" **"No!"** (= *1st No*)

Ask <u>one</u> of the "Not-Allowing-Questions": Can you allow your "Resistance" to your experience?
"No!" (= *2ⁿᵈ No*)

After the 2ⁿᵈ "No"
(in other words, after answering the
"Not-Allowing-Question" with "No")
→ Go back to the 1ˢᵗ Step of the Welcoming-Process and
ask yourself the Welcoming-Question once again.

1ˢᵗ Step - Welcoming: "I feel really sad that I lost so much money."
2ⁿᵈ Step - Allowing: Can you allow feeling sad that you lost so much money?" **Yes**

The 2ⁿᵈ "No" Rule:
After the 2ⁿᵈ "No" within the same Allowing-Step go back to
the 1ˢᵗ Step of the Welcoming-Process and ask yourself the
Welcoming-Question anew.

If you also answer your Not-Allowing-Question with *No* you *move on*, by *going back* to the Welcoming-Step and asking yourself the Welcoming-Question once again. In this way you ensure that the Welcoming-Process keeps moving and prevent yourself from getting stuck in the process. (For further and immediate visual clarification you can look at the Welcoming-Cycle on page 147)

A word of encouragement

This section on *not-allowing* or saying *No* to the content of your experience may seem a bit like a sidestep, and perhaps even a superfluous one. It is, however, central to the method. I assure you that once you have become familiar with the Not-Allowing-Questions, the purpose of this part of the process will become quite clear. *Understanding comes with doing the process* and even one or two attempts will demonstrate the energetic shift these questions bring about within your bodymind. All you need to do is continue reading and doing the exercises step-by-step. Before you know it, you will find yourself practicing the Welcoming-Process in your daily life. For now, just be patient with yourself and enjoy the ride!

When is the "Allowing-Step" complete?

> **When you have said "Yes" to *Allowing* the content of your experience, in the form of the *Allowing-Question* or *Not-Allowing-Question* and you have written down your answer, you have completed the Allowing-Step.**
> **Now you are ready to proceed to the 3rd Step of the Welcoming-Process.**

"Really ask yourself the Allowing-Question!"

It is important to note that there is no right or wrong answer to this question. You are neither compelled nor required to allow your experience, but you are asked to tell the truth about your willingness in the moment. Consciously and with genuine interest in hearing your own response, ask yourself the Allowing-Question, "Can you *really* allow the content of your experience?" Yes or No? Don't do it *mechanically* in a semi-conscious manner. The 2nd Step is not about *crossing off* the question in order to press ahead to the 3rd Step. Each step of the Welcoming-Process is designed to make it possible for you to become intimate with your experience. Therefore each step is equally important and meaningful and requires your full attention and conscious participation.

Take a moment, tune in and find out if you *truly* say *Yes* to allowing your experience. Maybe saying *No* to the Allowing-Question is the more honest, more authentic answer.

Participants who attend my Selflove-Training often have the idea that *allowing* is better than *not-allowing*. This is not so. *Yes* is not a better answer than *No*. What really matters is that you answer the Allowing-Question, as well as your Not-Allowing-Question, in integrity with your inner truth, the truth of your heart. That's it!

If you say: "Yes"
it means that you <u>can & do</u> give your *conscious consent* to allow
the content of your experience just as it is.

**If you say: "No" it means that you <u>cannot & don't</u>
give your *conscious consent* to *allow* the content of your
experience just as it is.**

The "safety valve" of the Welcoming-Process

Honoring your resistance, your "No" is an act of Selflove.

Saying *No* is your way to set a limit, uphold your boundary, and maintain your current state of being. The basic intention of *No* is to secure your need for *safety* and well-being. *No* respects and affirms your limits and your needs for boundaries, space, privacy, and protection. Your sense of safety constantly changes. On that score, your relationship with yourself is not all that different from a relationship with another: one day you long for a lot closeness and intimacy, and on another day you need a lot of *space* and time for yourself.

The Allowing-Step always gives you the freedom to say *No* and thus say *Yes* to your resistance. The process never forces you to *allow* an experience that you don't feel ready for. It is not only natural, it is totally okay to have resistance and feel aversion to certain contents of experience. It is also perfectly normal to need limits. You no longer have to be your ideal self and suffer from the stress of having to be more evolved than you really are. If some content of experience feels like *too much*—too scary, too intense, too uncomfortable, too risky—for you to *allow* just yet, give yourself permission to set an internal limit and simply say, *"No, I cannot allow it."* The simple act of *allowing* your limits and your resistances creates safety. You don't have to be any different than you are in any moment—that is the beauty of this practice! You are finally being *allowed* to be exactly as you are, and to feel exactly what you feel inside with a full range of openness and resistance to what you experience.

> **The possibility to say "No" to *allowing* the content of your experience, is an intentional element of the Welcoming-Process that ensures that you respect your own limits and your need for safety, which is a safeguard against *allowing* an experience that feels too overwhelming in any given moment.**

The option of saying, *No* to allowing the content of your experience represents the *safety valve* of the Welcoming-Process. You might be confronted with a situation that brings up enormous grief or fear. You might choose to do the Welcoming-Process and as you come to the 2nd Step and ask the

Allowing-Question, you may realize that the grief or the fear feels too over-whelming to allow at that moment. In this case you would say simply, *"No, I cannot allow this enormous grief / fear"*, and thus make use of the safety valve. Then, you would move on to the next step and ask yourself one of the Not-Allowing-Questions, for example: *"Can you allow your resistance?"* This step will likely come easy and as you allow your resistance to "what is" in the moment you will realize what a loving act it is to respect your limits and your need for boundaries. Learning to say *No* to allowing your here and now experi-ence is crucial in cultivating the Art of Selflove.

**Saying "No" from the bottom of your heart is truly saying "Yes"
to yourself.**

THE COMPLETE FORMULA FOR THE
"ALLOWING-STEP"

---

1. **Write down the Allowing-Question:**
    "Can you allow your experience?"

2. **Write down Your Answer: "Yes" or "No"**
    If your answer is "Yes" then the Allowing-Step is complete!

3. **If your answer is "No" ask yourself one of the 3
    Not-Allowing-Questions & write it down your answer.**

3A. **If your answer is "Yes" then the Allowing-Step is complete!**

3B. **If your answer is "No" (i.e. the 2ⁿᵈ "No")**
    **then go back to the 1ˢᵗ Step of the Welcoming-Process
    and ask yourself the Welcoming-Question again...**

    ... & just keep going...

    That's it!

EXERCISE - BECOME FAMILIAR WITH THE ALLOWING-STEP

As this is only a preparatory exercise to become familiar with the Allowing-Step make sure that you do this exercise when you are in a *good space* and at ease with yourself.

Practice the Welcoming-Step & Allowing-Step:

1. Write in your Selflove-Journal, *"Practicing the Welcoming- & Allowing-Steps"*
2. Practice the Welcoming- & Allowing-Steps with ten different contents of experience and number each of them from 1-10.

Example: 1.
1. 1st Step: Welcoming: "I feel calm inside."
   2nd Step: Allowing: Can you allow feeling calm inside? Yes!

Keep going until you have completely *Welcomed & Allowed* ten different experiences.

To make this exercise easier for yourself, I invite you to look once more at the previous ten Welcoming & Allowing examples on page 115 & 116, and the *complete formula of the Allowing-Step* on page 124. Browsing through the book and looking up the information you need will help you memorize each of the steps and become familiar the Welcoming-Process.

"ALLOWING" YOUR EXPERIENCE DOES NOT MEAN "ACTING OUT"

There is a world of difference between *allowing* the content of your experience and *expressing* it. Allowing your experience simply means that you say *Yes* to experiencing the content inside your bodymind. It does not mean that you are going to *act out* your experience in the external world. To clarify this significant point, let's look at a practical example taken from a Welcoming-Session.

1st Step: Welcoming: "I want to hit him and yell at him."
2nd Step: Allowing: Can you allow wanting to hit him and yell at him? Yes.

Allowing *wanting to hit him and yell at him* by saying *Yes* and *allowing your wanting* does not mean that you are really going to hit and yell at the other person. When you say, *"Yes!"* you are simply allowing yourself to experience your *wanting to act out* internally, in your bodymind. Therefore allowing an experience and acting out the actual experience is not the same. Once you have completed your Welcoming-Session, you can still decide if you will choose to express what you have just experienced inside, and if so what part and how.

SELF-CONTAINMENT IS A NATURAL "BYPRODUCT" OF THE ALLOWING-STEP

***Self-containment* is your ability to *allow* the content of your experience, without *having to act it out* automatically based on your habitual behavior & reaction patterns.**

Self-containment is the *third way* of dealing with your internal experiences. If you *contain* your experience, you don't repress it, nor do you express it right away. You can imagine that inside of you is a *container*, an inner vessel or cauldron that has the ability to contain all of your experiences, no matter how exciting or challenging the actual content is. The consistent practice of the Welcoming-Process, especially the Allowing-Step, keeps expanding, strengthening, and solidifying your *inner container* which enables you to contain the multifaceted contents of experience. Increasing self-containment gives you an enormous freedom since you are less and less controlled by external circumstances and the reactive behavior pattern of the little-i. The Allowing-Step gives you a new option: to contain your inner experience, enabling you to choose if you really want to express your internal experience (what you sense, need, feel, think, etc.), and if yes, in what way, what part of it, when, and with whom.

The more you learn to intentionally contain your experience with the Allowing-Step, the stronger and bigger your inner container grows and with it your *love-ability**, your ability to love yourself with your here and now experience or another with her/his experience. With practice what you currently go through, what the actual content of your experience is, will matter less and less, you will just *welcome & allow* it, and thus relate to it in a conscious and loving way.

"ALLOWING" IS A PATH OF CULTIVATING
A LOVING ATTITUDE

Allowing **is an all-embracing & all-loving attitude.**
It knows no resistance and therefore embraces all resistance.
Nothing, no experience, no content, is *too dirty,* *too ugly,*
or *too bad* to be received, contained & transformed in its
all-loving embrace.

Simply asking yourself the Allowing-Question—*Can you allow your here and now experience? —automatically* cultivates a loving attitude towards yourself. The actual question naturally invites a loving way of relating to yourself and the content of your experience.

Imagine that you have a sacred temple inside of you, a *temple of Selflove.* The entrance hall of the temple, consisting of a large, wide-open portal, stands for the Welcoming-Step that *welcomes* all of your experiences. Every experience is invited to come into the open reception chamber, into the presence of your conscious awareness. No experience is refused, rejected, criticized, or attacked. Nothing has to be any different than it is. Whatever your experience is, it is being *welcomed* and consciously recognized as it is. Once the content of your experience has *checked-in* and passed through the 1st Step of the process, it is led to the second chamber of the Selflove temple, the hall of the Allowing-Step. There you can see a huge, round, light-filled basin held and contained by two arms with interlaced fingers. This is the *allowing-vessel,* your inner container, which embraces and contains all of your experiences with its loving attitude. Once you say *Yes* to allowing the content of your experience,

---

*The ability to love or to *welcome & allow* whatever the content of your experience is.

it plunges into the allowing-vessel where it is fully held, and fully *allowed* to be just as it is.

**"When you allow something to be exactly the way it is,
it allows you to be."**
Ariel & Shya Kane

THE ACTUAL-ALLOWING HAPPENS BY ITSELF — *AUTOMATICALLY*

**"The first step toward change is acceptance.
Once you accept yourself, you open the door to change.
That's all you have to do.
Change is not something you do, it's something you allow."**
Will Garcia

The *Actual-Allowing* happens when all of you, your conscious mind and your body, your whole bodymind, says *Yes* internally to *fully Allowing* the content of your here & now experience".

The *actual-allowing* happens by itself. You cannot force it, nor can you make it happen with your will. The actual-allowing is not a voluntary action; it is something that comes about spontaneously, much like a yawn. The Allowing-Question is the preliminary procedure that leads up to the moment of the actual-allowing. You can compare it to the process of yawning. Let's assume you deliberately choose to yawn. Usually you initiate yawning by closing your eyes, which assists you in bringing your attention inside your body. Then you open your mouth widely and alter your breathing in a way that produces the characteristic yawning sound. Meanwhile you stay in this *surrendered* state or position and wait until the *actual yawning response* takes over and leads you into a *full blown yawning experience* with its typical body-signals and body-sensations, for example the intense stretching and relaxation movement of your mouth, jaw, and throat muscles, as well as the profound inhalation and exhalation.

A similar phenomenon happens when you do the Allowing-Step. After you intentionally say *Yes* to allowing your here and now experience, you remain fully aware, in this receptive and open state, until your bodymind *says Yes internally to allowing* the content of your experience. Once your bodymind says *Yes* to allowing the content of your experience the actual-allowing automatically takes place.

There is an intimate connection between happiness and allowing, which is why this step is so important in cultivating the Art of Selflove.

"Happiness is a function of accepting what is."
Werner Erhard

"Happiness can exist only in acceptance."
Denis De Rougemont

Now, you have received all the necessary information to go on to the next chapter, the 3rd and final step of the Welcoming-Process, called Noticing-the-Bodyshift.

CHAPTER 9

"NOTICING-THE-BODYSHIFT"
- The 3rd Step of the Welcoming-Process

WHAT IS THE "BODYSHIFT"?

> **The "Bodyshift" is an involuntary physical change that occurs automatically in the moment of the Actual-Allowing.**

THIS third and final step of the Welcoming-Process gives you physical feedback in the form of a bodily signal that is a tangible confirmation of the whole-body nature of this method. *Noticing-the-Bodyshift* is not an intellectual exercise or heady process, but a full bodymind experience that anchors your awareness in your physical body right in the moment. The bodyshift itself is a clear *body signal* (a sudden inhalation, strong exhalation, yawn, or giggle, for example) that evidences the actual-allowing that has come about within your bodymind. You cannot make it happen voluntarily; it is a spontaneous phenomenon that happens beyond your volitional control. When your bodymind *internally* says *Yes* to allowing the content of your experience then a clearly noticeable change, the bodyshift, automatically occurs within your physical body.

The bodyshift, which is brought about by the self-regulation of your bodymind, is the physical confirmation that the content of your experience has been *fully allowed*. Noticing-the-Bodyshift is a *self-empowering feedback mechanism* that informs you that your bodymind has *fully allowed* your here and now experience, and that *the process is working.*

Noticing-the-Bodyshift is the *feedback-step* of the
Welcoming-Process that lets you know in the form of a clear,
spontaneous body signal that the *Actual-Allowing* has happened;
in other words that your bodymind has *fully allowed*
the content of your experience.

THE TWO MAJOR BODYSHIFTS

A spontaneous change or *shift* in the *way you breathe* is a
primary bodyshift. All the other *shifts* in your body are *secondary
bodyshifts.*

Bodyshifts that cause a change in the way you breathe are *Primary Bodyshifts;* these are the most common and the easiest to perceive. All other *shifts* that do not directly involve your breathing are *Secondary Bodyshifts.*

Primary Bodyshifts

- **Automatic, involuntary changes in the way you breathe, for example: you suddenly inhale or exhale more deeply/slowly from your chest and/or belly region**
- **Unintentional sounds involving your breathing, like giggling, laughing, sighing, moaning, burping, etc.**
- **Yawning**

Secondary Bodyshifts

- **Relaxation – Changes in your muscle tone**
- **Involuntary body movements, such as spontaneous smiling, trembling, shaking, tingling, streaming sensations, etc.**
- **Change in temperature – either warmer or cooler**
- **Change in weight – you feel lighter or heavier**
- **Change in sense of space – you feel more spacious or more compact/solid**
- **Change of presence – you feel more present in your body or in parts of it**
- **Sounds in the body, such as gurgling, grumbling, etc.**

EXAMPLES OF BODYSHIFTS TAKEN FROM DIFFERENT WELCOMING-SESSIONS:

- "I just took a deep breath."
- "A sigh came out."
- "I realize that I just started breathing into my belly."
- "My breathing just calmed down."
- "Both my shoulders came down a bit, relaxed."
- "My hands are getting warmer."
- "My body, and especially my arms, feel lighter".
- "I have more space in my chest."
- "My breathing feels more flowing."
- "My legs feel suddenly more solid, more compact."
- "My gut is making a funny gurgling sound."
- "I feel more present in my body."

In the beginning, you will need a quiet place and intentional focus to actually bring your awareness into your body and perceive a bodyshift. This is normal, and yet most people are surprised at how clear and unambiguous the shift is once they slow down and begin to notice their body-sensations. With regular practice, it will become second nature to you. A bodyshift is sometimes quite subtle, yet it has a distinct and satisfying quality that accompanies the spontaneous change within your body.

All bodyshifts, primary or secondary, are equally valid and equally valuable. As you are learning to notice your bodyshifts pay foremost attention to your breathing, since changes in the way you breathe are generally the easiest to perceive. No matter how subtle or insignificant the bodyshift might seem, any bodyshift you notice is a *good* one.

A GENERAL BODYMIND-PRINCIPLE

**Whenever there is a change in your mind,
there is a change in the way you breathe, a primary Bodyshift.
Whenever there is a change in the way you breathe,
there is a change in the mind, a *Mindshift*.**

By regularly Noticing-the-Bodyshift you will begin to see that whatever happens in your mind or psyche is *reflected* in your physical body as well. For example: let's say you find yourself worrying about your finances. Tuning into your body, you sense that your stomach is tensing up and your breathing has become fast and shallow. Suddenly your best friend calls to say she wants to treat you to dinner at your favorite restaurant and you observe a sense of elation move through you. It's not just that your mind has opened up to receive this gift, your whole body gets a boost of energy. Noticing-the-Bodyshift will make this intimate connection between your body and your mind ever more obvious to you. Then the term bodymind will no longer be just a concept, but a living experience.

A quick reminder:

Since the Welcoming-Process is a three-step method, you need to make sure that you have completed the 1st & 2nd Step before going on to the 3rd Step, Noticing-the-Bodyshift.

How do you "Notice the Bodyshift"?

1.
Bring your awareness into your physical body
&
Be attentive to your body-sensations and body signals
- Focusing on your breathing is the easiest! -

2.
Simply observe
&
Notice the Bodyshift
as the *Actual-Allowing* occurs
(For example: a change in your breathing)

The moment you sense a clear, distinct change,
or *shift* in your body, you *notice the Bodyshift*.

3.
Write down your answer or Bodyshift !
(For example: deep inhalation or long exhalation)

One Bodyshift is *Enough!*

You <u>only</u> need to "Notice <u>one</u> Bodyshift",
a primary or secondary Bodyshift, in order to complete
the 3rd Step of the Welcoming-Process.

While you may experience more than one bodyshift—perhaps you yawn and then notice your shoulders drop an inch—one such shift is enough to complete this third step of the process. Even a subtle secondary shift is enough to signal that your body has responded to the Allowing-Step and fully allowed the experience.

When is "Noticing-the-Bodyshift" complete?

> **When you have written down the kind of Bodyshift that you have just noticed you have completed the 3rd Step of the Welcoming-Process.**

I have said it before, and yet this point bears repeating here. Putting down on paper each of these 3 simple steps is absolutely crucial since the full power of the Welcoming-Process—especially when you are dealing with a highly charged emotional issue—can only unfold if you do the process in a written way. So, do not skip over this important element of the process since it is also the foundation to going through each of the 3 steps *just in your head* when you are in the middle of stressful situation and really in need of relating to yourself in a conscious and loving way. Remember, you are building a new skill and that takes practice and repetition, and writing down each step is the basis to mastering this process and thus the Art of Selflove.

10 Practical examples of Noticing-the-Bodyshift

Below are 10 different examples of what people have experienced when Noticing-the-Bodyshift. They have been drawn from actual Welcoming-Sessions:

1. 1st Step - Welcoming: "I can just be myself because I follow my inner truth."
   2nd Step - Allowing: Can you allow just being yourself? Yes.
   3rd Step - Notice the Bodyshift as the Actual-Allowing occurs: Deep breath and yawning

2. 1st Step - Welcoming: "I am tired of giving and supporting."
   2nd Step - Allowing: Can you allow being tired of giving and supporting? Yes.
   3rd Step - Notice the Bodyshift as the Actual-Allowing occurs: Deep inhalation

3. 1st Step - Welcoming: "I feel unworthy."
   2nd Step - Allowing: Can you allow feeling unworthy? <u>No.</u>
   Ask <u>One</u> of the Not-Allowing-Questions: Can you allow your Not-Allowing? Yes.
   3rd Step - Notice the Bodyshift as the Actual-Allowing occurs: Intense yawning

4. 1st Step - Welcoming: "I long for a really special partner."
   2nd Step - Allowing: Can you allow this longing for a special partner? Yes.
   3rd Step - Notice the Bodyshift as the Actual-Allowing occurs: Deep exhalation and deeper breathing

5. 1st Step - Welcoming: "I feel some fear and some excitement."
   2nd Step - Allowing: Can you allow feeling some fear and some excitement? Yes.
   3rd Step - Notice the Bodyshift as the Actual-Allowing occurs: Deep Breath and smiling

6. 1st Step - Welcoming: "I want to be the best – stand out and be loved."
   2nd Step - Allowing: Can you allow wanting to be the best, to stand out and to be loved? <u>No.</u>
   Ask <u>One</u> of the Not-Allowing-Questions: Can you allow your Resistance? Yes.
   3rd Step - Notice the Bodyshift as the Actual-Allowing occurs: Deep breath and relaxation in my neck

7. 1st Step - Welcoming: "I am a good human being even if I don't produce."
   2nd Step - Allowing: Can you allow being a good human being? Yes.
   3rd Step - Notice the Bodyshift as the Actual-Allowing occurs: Deep Breath and relaxation in my belly

8.   1st Step - Welcoming: "This process takes my fear away."
     2nd Step - Allowing: Can you allow that this process takes away your fear? Yes.
     3rd Step - Notice the Bodyshift as the Actual-Allowing occurs: More calmness in my body and (a few seconds later) **intense yawning**

9.   1st Step - Welcoming: "I want this pain to go away!"
     2nd Step - Allowing: Can you allow wanting this pain to go away? Yes.
     3rd Step - Notice the Bodyshift as the Actual-Allowing occurs: Yawning

10. 1st Step - Welcoming: "I think back on similarly painful situations."
     2nd Step - Allowing: Can you allow thinking back on similarly painful situations? No.
     Ask <u>One</u> of the Not-Allowing-Questions: Can you allow your Resistance? Yes
     3rd Step - Notice the Bodyshift as the Actual-Allowing occurs: A deep sigh

WHAT DO YOU DO AFTER YOU HAVE "NOTICED THE BODYSHIFT"?

After you have *Noticed the Bodyshift* and written down your answer, continue the process by going back to the beginning and repeating each of the 3 basic steps of the Welcoming-Process: the *Welcoming-Step*, the *Allowing-Step*, & *Noticing-the-Bodyhift-Step*.

Once you have noticed the bodyshift and written down your answer you have completed the 3rd and final Step of the Welcoming-Process. But this is not the end of the actual process. The Welcoming-Process is a *cyclical process*, which means that you keep repeating the three steps over and over again. The power of the Welcoming-Process lies to a large degree in the ongoing repetition of each of the three basic steps.

Further details about how the three steps work together, how you do a complete Welcoming-Session and how many times you repeat the three steps until a session is complete will be explained in the next chapter.

For now, all that you need to know is this: after you have completed the 3rd Step, Noticing-the-Bodyshift, go back to the beginning and once again move through each of the 3 basic steps while writing it down as illustrated in the above examples.

How long does it take for the Bodyshift to occur?

The emergence of the bodyshift is an individual phenomenon. In general, people tend to experience the bodyshift within 10 seconds of answering the Allowing-Question or Not-Allowing-Question with *Yes*. This is a general guideline, however, under some circumstances it might take 10 to 20 seconds and in rare situations up to 30 seconds or more. Usually in the beginning, while you are still finding out how the Welcoming-Process works it takes more time because you might *miss* the first bodyshift and only notice the second or third one. Also, it is likely new for you to pay conscious attention to your body-sensations. Like any relationship, your relationship with your body grows over time.

Remember: the bodyshift comes about naturally and spontaneously. It cannot be willed, forced, or pushed in any way. The actual-allowing can only be *allowed*. Once it occurs, then the bodyshift is the natural result. So, please, be patient with yourself since you are learning a totally new skill. Don't worry if you don't perceive the bodyshift in the beginning. With practice you will notice it!

The more you practice the Welcoming-Process the easier it will be for you to Notice the Bodyshift.

Exercise: become familiar with Noticing-the-Bodyshift

In this exercise you will have the opportunity to experience what you have read about Noticing-the-Bodyshift. This exercise is not yet an entire Welcoming-Session although you will go through each of the 3 Steps of the Welcoming-Process. The intention of this exercise is primarily to learn to notice the bodyshift, in the moment when the actual-allowing occurs. Make sure that you are in a rather positive and relaxed state when you do this exercise.

1. Begin by writing the following heading in your Selflove-Journal: *Practicing the 3 Steps of the Welcoming-Process*
2. Do the Welcoming-Step
3. Do the Allowing-Step—keep going until you have answered the Allowing Question or Not-Allowing-Question with *Yes*
4. Right after you said *Yes*—bring your awareness into your body and be attentive to your body-sensations & body signals.
5. *Simply observe and notice the bodyshift* as the actual-allowing occurs
6. Write down what kind of bodyshift you noticed
7. Keep repeating points 2 – 6 until you have gone through each of the 3 Steps of the Welcoming-Process 10 times. Number each completed section from 1-10, as you have seen in the previous examples.

On page 136 – 138 you will find the exact visual outline of how to do the above exercise.

After completing this exercise you will be more familiar with Noticing-the-Bodyshift. On occasion, you will not perceive a bodyshift at all. How can this be and what do you do then?

"I notice no Bodyshift!"

Sometimes people who are learning the Welcoming-Process say, "This time no bodyshift emerged!" or "There has been no bodyshift." The reason for this is that the bodyshift happened so quickly that it bypassed conscious awareness.

It is very common for the bodyshift to occur right away after you've said,

"Yes" (I can allow my experience...) or while you are still in the process of writing down the Allowing-Question. As you are writing, *"Can you allow this feeling..." internally* your bodymind already says, *"Yes,"* and therefore the actual-allowing, the bodyshift, happens before you write down the Allowing-Question or Not-Allowing-Question. Then by the time you say, "Yes, I can allow it" the bodyshift has already occurred and is *long gone.* The other reason you might not notice a bodyshift is simply because your conscious mind is not yet attuned to the somatic level of its body-sensations and simply doesn't perceive it. Again, this takes time. Many of us have spent decades living in our heads; learning to inhabit the body more fully and catch its signals will come and—trust me on this—it will be a very satisfying discovery.

WHAT DO YOU DO IF YOU "NOTICE NO BODYSHIFT"?

If it seems to you that there is really no bodyshift happening within a minute after you've said, *"Yes, I can allow my here and now experience,"* then do the following:

Ask yourself, "Can you allow the fact that you don't perceive a Bodyshift?"

It is most likely that allowing the above experience will automatically bring about a bodyshift.

If you still don't get a bodyshift simply move on, return to the 1st Step of the Welcoming-Process, and ask yourself the Welcoming-Question. Just be gentle with yourself; you are learning a new skill. Once you notice the first bodyshift, a second one will follow and eventually *sensing bodyshifts* will become very easy for you. If you occasionally *miss a bodyshift* simply ask yourself, "Can you allow the fact that you don't perceive a bodyshift?" and continue the process.

Sometimes, after you have said, "yes" to allowing the content of your experience, you feel an inner urge to take a deep breath, to make a sigh, to yawn, or to stretch your body.

By following this inner urge you automatically invite the Bodyshift to occur.

Multiple Bodyshifts

Occasionally you might notice more than one bodyshift. In this case you have *multiple bodyshifts*. Often they occur one after another, like beads on a string, and at other times they all happen simultaneously. Multiple bodyshifts consist of two or more bodyshifts. For example, you may take a deep breath, then relax your left shoulder, feel a sensation of warmth in the upper body, and then notice that you are smiling. It does not matter if you notice the first or the last bodyshift in a sequence of multiple bodyshifts. It is important that you notice at least one bodyshift, because this completes the 3rd Step of the Welcoming-Process.

You might also experience an *extended* or *ongoing* bodyshift. For example, you keep yawning several times and it seems to go on for a while. This is totally fine. Just follow the wisdom of your bodymind, since it knows exactly what it needs to do in order to balance itself.

Two examples of multiple Bodyshifts taken from Welcoming-Sessions:

- "A deep breath fills up my whole chest and shortly after I begin to yawn."
- "My jaw is *thawing up* - it becomes softer. Then I notice a deep inhalation followed by a sigh." (It is quite common to exhale in the form of a sigh.)

Yawning is a powerful Bodyshift

Yawning is a very safe and powerful way that your bodymind discharges old tensions in order to transform, harmonize, and neutralize old blockages.

Do you remember ever having seen a film of a huge male lion lying on his belly and opening his mouth as wide as he can in order to allow a great yawn to emerge? The lion is fully present, totally aware, and enjoying the pleasurable *ripple-sensation* that moves through each fiber of his body. Unfortunately, *yawning* in the presence of another person is considered somewhat impolite in our culture. This is largely due to the assumption that a yawn means boredom or tiredness, when in fact science has found no such link associated with the yawn. What we do know about yawns is that they are contagious and they occur in most vertebrates—reptiles , fish, birds, and mammals. The following excerpts from the article, *"The incredible, communicable yawn"* confirm some of my own discoveries on the effect of yawning: "In fact, one function of yawning is its importance in changing behavioral states." Furthermore, "According to psychologist Olivier Walusinski, yawning is part of introspectiveness, or sensitivity to events happening within the body." And finally, "....yawning resets the mental self-image, thus increasing arousal and self-awareness."*1

I have found that yawns almost always accompany some kind of transitional moment, thought, or emotion. In other words, yawning is your body's way of saying, "Okay, we have integrated this experience... what's next?"

Once you consciously get into the *full-blown yawning experience* initiated by the Welcoming-Process you will begin to thoroughly enjoy it. Especially take note of its relaxing *aftereffect*. Although I specifically emphasize the powerful effect of yawning, this does not mean it is superior to the other forms the bodyshift might take. All bodyshifts are equally important.

"I feel *yawning* is dissolving old tensions in my body."
Siegbert K., a practitioner of the
Welcoming-Process

A fun game to play is trying to make another person yawn. I used to play it with my grandmother until she begged me to stop. Enjoy and explore *yawning* with the curiosity of a child.

All Bodyshifts are equally precious and important.
All that matters for the Welcoming-Process is that you notice
<u>one</u> Bodyshift at a time.

"Noticing-the-Bodyshift"
is a path of embodying Selflove

Noticing-the-Bodyshift is a path to becoming deeply centered and present in your body.

The 3rd Step, Noticing-the-Bodyshift, intentionally anchors your awareness in your body by consistently bringing your attention back to the sensations and signals it is giving you. In this way you become ever more fully present and centered in your physical body. The Welcoming-Process is a *body-centered-process* since it engages the *neocortex*, the conscious part of your brain, as well as the instinctive, body-centered part of your brain, called the reptilian brain.

The reptilian brain represents the *inner animal*, the primitive side of you that speaks a non-verbal, instinctive language. The animal in you communicates through body-sensations, body signals, gestures, and body postures. Pleasant or comfortable body sensations, such as deep breathing or relaxed muscle tone, let you know that the animal within you feels safe, at ease. On the other hand, unpleasant or uncomfortable body-sensations, such as quick and shallow chest breathing or the tensing up of certain muscles, indicate that your inner animal feels threatened, no longer safe, and stressed.

Noticing-the-Bodyshift is a practice of centering yourself in your physical body that enables you to get to know your inner animal and hear its intuitive messages. You might call them gut feelings or a sense of inner knowing; all of these will be amplified when you begin to attend to the bodyshift.

Noticing-the-Bodyshift, the 3rd Step of the Welcoming-Process, *anchors* your Selflove, the art of loving yourself, in your body.

This concludes the information on Noticing-the-Bodyshift. In the next chapter I will introduce to you the *Welcoming-Cycle,* which will answer any of your open questions regarding the application of the 3 Steps of the Welcoming-Process.

CHAPTER 10

The Heart of the Welcoming-Process

"You have noticed that everything an Indian does is in a circle
and that is because the power of the world always works in
circles, and everything tries to be round...
The sky is round, and I have heard that the earth is round
like a ball, and so are the stars.
The wind, in its greatest power, whirls.
Even the seasons form a great circle in their changing
and always come back again to where they were.
The life of a man is a circle from childhood
to childhood, and so it is in everything
where power moves."
Black Elk, Lakota Medicine Man

THE Welcoming-Process is a powerful circular system. The *hidden power* behind this method lies in the cyclical and continual application of the 3 basic steps. Any life issue or theme that you work with will begin to transform and harmonize automatically as you take yourself through a Welcoming-Session.

THE WELCOMING-CYCLE

The Welcoming-Cycle is the *heart* or central technique of the Welcoming-Process.

The diagram below represents the essential technique of the Welcoming-Process. This graphic illustration will help you understand how the 3 steps of the process work together as a circular system. The Welcoming-Cycle is a simplified outline and summary of all the necessary information that you need to do a complete Welcoming-Session for yourself.

The Welcoming-Cycle™

Welcoming
Ask the Welcoming-Question:
"What are you experiencing right now?"

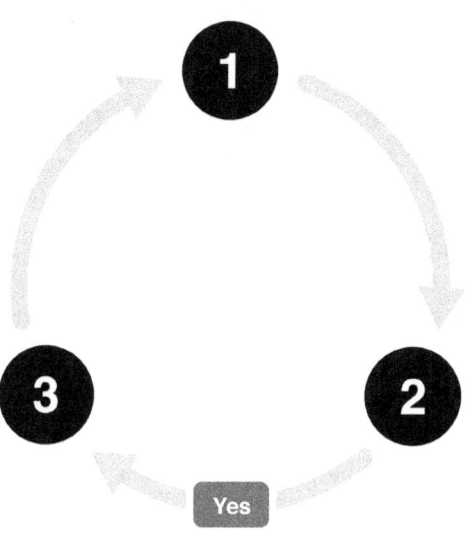

Noticing-the-Bodyshift
Bring awareness into your body:
*Observe your body-sensations &
Notice the Bodyshift*

Allowing
Ask the Allowing-Question:
"Can you allow your experience?"

No

**Ask the
Not-Allowing-Question:**
*Can you allow your No /
Not-Allowing / Resistance?*

No

**Go back to
Restart the Welcoming-Cycle**

> **Going through each of the 3 Steps of the Welcoming-Process completes <u>one</u> Welcoming-Cycle.**

THE PLATEAU PHASE

In the course of a Welcoming-Session, when a content of experience emerges that you feel fully at ease with you have reached a *plateau*.

Normally you start a Welcoming-Session by choosing a specific issue, called the *session theme*. A session theme could be stress at work, money worries, relationship conflict, feeling moody, or some other situation that causes an emotional upset. A session theme usually begins with an uncomfortable or somewhat disturbing content of experience. With each Welcoming-Cycle the original quality of the session theme automatically transforms and eventually harmonizes itself, thus bringing you to the plateau. Reaching a plateau is an indication that you have come to a point in the session where you feel okay with your here and now experience. Typically accompanied by a sense of ease, inner peace, and wellbeing, the plateau is the *resting* and *relaxation phase* of the Welcoming-Process.

"I know I have reached a plateau when I feel okay with my here & now experience."
Raven – a practitioner of the Welcoming-Process

The plateau is the peaceful resting phase that you reach automatically after you have gone through a certain number of Welcoming-Cycles.

WHAT DO YOU DO WHEN YOU REACH A PLATEAU?

The plateau is a time for *orienting & checking-in*.

When you reach a plateau it is time to pause and take a break from your Welcoming-Session. Relax and bring your attention back to the outer world by looking at the shapes, colors, and structures of the objects in your environment. This allows you to *orient* yourself—to get reacquainted with your surroundings—while you adjust to the changes that have occurred in your overall state. Orienting automatically invites your nervous system to bridge the perception of your inner and outer world, thus creating a natural balance between the two. In this sense the plateau is not only a resting phase, but also an integration phase that gives you an opportunity to incorporate the *harmonizing aftereffects* of the Welcoming-Process. Giving yourself enough time to look around and orient yourself is vital because the process involves an intense inner focus that causes you to disengage from the exterior world. Once you feel fully *oriented*, fully aware of your outer world and well grounded in your bodymind, it is time to check-in with yourself and decide whether to carry on with the session or end it at this point. Your physical body can help you make this decision. If your body begins to feel uneasy or to tighten up when you think of continuing the session, then you know that this is your body's way of signaling you to conclude the session for now. Your body signals will become more obvious in time; all that is required is a willingness to listen and act on the signals.

It is crucial to respect your limits, listen to your body signals, and not push yourself beyond what feels right. In this way you always give yourself enough time and space to integrate the changes that occur in a Welcoming-Session. Remember that your bodymind has its own innate intelligence and knows exactly how much transformation it can handle at a time.

When you reach a plateau...

... you take a break, lean back, look around, and *orient* to your environment. Once you feel fully centered, you check-in with your body and decide if it feels right to end your Welcoming-Session or to go on by starting a new Welcoming-Cycle.

ORIENTING: CONSCIOUSLY FOLLOW YOUR EYES

To get a better understanding of what *orienting* is, imagine a dog walking through tall grass in a meadow. All the dog does is follow the interesting smells his nose picks up. In the same way, let your eyes wander around by letting them look at whatever they are drawn to in your environment. Instead of directing your eyes or having them focus intentionally on a specific object, just observe how your eyes enjoy roaming about.

> **"Orienting is a different way of looking. It is not looking at things; it is being present with things... This way of looking helps me to integrate my inner experience with the outer world."**
> Roger M. – a practitioner of the Welcoming-Process

In order to do an entire Welcoming-Session it is important that you keep going until you reach a plateau. Going through as many cycles as you need to reach a plateau is a crucial *safety-valve* of the Welcoming-Process. This ensures that you only bring the session to a close when you are in a well-oriented, well-grounded, and well-balanced state of being.

The Plateau Rule:

In order to do a complete written Welcoming-Session you always go on with the Welcoming-Process until you reach a plateau.

LEARNING TO RECOGNIZE THE PLATEAU

During this initial phase when you are still becoming familiar with the steps of the process, you may not recognize the moment when you reach a plateau. That is to be expected; your learning curve will be unique to you. Be patient. Once you have a sense of how the cycle goes, the plateau phase will become more palpable. Sometimes it is very clear that you have reached a plateau while in other sessions it will be less obvious. In the course of an extended Welcoming-Session you will experience multiple plateaus. So don't worry if you miss a plateau, there will be another one if you keep going and take yourself through further Welcoming-Cycles.

Read through the complete Welcoming-Session examples in this chapter and the ones that follow to get a clear understanding of what a plateau is and, more importantly, what it feels like. The session below will give you an example of how the process leads you through several plateaus that you can then number like this: 1st plateau… 2nd plateau… 3rd plateau… etc.

A complete Welcoming-Session

The following session integrates the theoretical information on the Welcoming-Process that you have read so far. I recommend reading the session with your full attention in order to get a clear understanding, as well as a deeper feeling, for the process as a whole. I intentionally chose to present a psychologically intense session theme right from the start so you can see that this method can help you move through highly charged emotional issues. Once you have mastered this process and made it part of how you relate to life, even quite challenging contents of experience can be met with grace and ease.

Lou embraces her anxiety

Lou came to see me to deal with her anxiety about going into the hospital. She was scheduled to have major surgery in two weeks and was having trouble sleeping because she was so worried about the operation. It was not her first time going under anesthesia, but she was terrified that something could go wrong. Lou had some experience with the Welcoming-Process but was finding it difficult to work through a complete Welcoming-Session by herself, so she asked me to guide her through the entire process.

Session theme: Scheduled operation and sensation of pressure on chest

1. 1st Step - Welcoming: **"I remember earlier operations."**
   2nd Step - Allowing: Can you allow **remembering these earlier operations? Yes**
   3rd Step - Notice the Bodyshift as the Actual-Allowing occurs: **A sigh**

2. 1ˢᵗ Step - Welcoming: **"I feel grief."**
   2ⁿᵈ Step - Allowing: Can you allow **this feeling of grief?** Yes.
   3ʳᵈ Step - Notice the Bodyshift as the Actual-Allowing occurs:
   Breathing becomes faster

3. 1ˢᵗ Step - Welcoming: **"I am far away from everything."**
   2ⁿᵈ Step - Allowing: Can you allow **being far away from everything? Yes.**
   3ʳᵈ Step - Notice the Bodyshift as the Actual-Allowing occurs:
   Yawning

4. 1ˢᵗ Step - Welcoming: **"It feels lighter in the chest."**
   2ⁿᵈ Step - Allowing: Can you allow **feeling lighter in the chest? Yes.**
   3ʳᵈ Step - Notice the Bodyshift as the Actual-Allowing occurs: **More yawning**

1ˢᵗ Plateau: "**Right now I am glad that my chest feels lighter.**"
Lou realizes that she has reached a first plateau. She begins to orient herself while looking around the room. As she becomes fully centered and grounded in the here and now, she decides to continue the process.

5. 1ˢᵗ Step - Welcoming: **"I feel more courage."**
   2ⁿᵈ Step - Allowing: Can you allow **feeling more courage? Yes**
   3ʳᵈ Step - Notice the Bodyshift as the Actual-Allowing occurs:
   Yawning

6. 1ˢᵗ Step - Welcoming: **"I feel more relaxed inside."**
   2ⁿᵈ Step - Allowing: Can you allow **feeling more relaxed inside? Yes**
   3ʳᵈ Step - Notice the Bodyshift as the Actual-Allowing occurs: **Deep breath & more yawning**

7. 1ˢᵗ Step - Welcoming: **"I feel more relaxation in my chest."**
   2ⁿᵈ Step - Allowing: Can you allow **feeling more relaxation in your chest? Yes**
   3ʳᵈ Step - Notice the Bodyshift as the Actual-Allowing occurs: **Yawning**

8. 1ˢᵗ Step - Welcoming: **"My fear goes away."**
   2ⁿᵈ Step - Allowing: Can you allow **your fear going away? Yes**
   3ʳᵈ Step - Notice the Bodyshift as the Actual-Allowing occurs: **More yawning & body calms down**

2ⁿᵈ <u>Plateau</u>: **"I'm feeling that I can look forward to the operation now. It feels like a liberation. I see myself being healthy. Right now, I feel very centered. I am breathing from the center of my body unlike before when I seemed to be hovering somewhere outside my body. My belly and chest feel softer... I feel peaceful. This is a good place for me to end the session."**

Session time: 15 minutes

THE SNOWBALL EFFECT

Each Welcoming-Cycle builds upon the previous one, as does each Welcoming-Session. The Welcoming-Process is a cumulative, ever deepening and ever expanding process. With each session you cultivate the Art of Selflove and ever more fully face and embrace the whole reality of being human, rather than avoiding your experience. This can be a radical departure from the state of confused overwhelm or numbed-out denial that passes for coping in a demanding world. Every time you go through a new Welcoming-Cycle, you learn to relate to your here and now experience in an ever more conscious and loving way. Imagine a snowball that grows ever bigger and more powerful with each additional going round. Your ability to love yourself and accept life on its own terms grows in the same way each time you go through a new cycle.

SELF-REGULATION

**"Since the psyche is a self-regulating system, just as the body
is, the regulating counteraction will always develop in the
unconscious."**
C. G. Jung

Self-regulation is an intelligent process of your bodymind that automatically transforms any content of your experience that you welcome & allow. The same way your physical body has a self-regulating mechanism called *homeostasis,* your psyche has its own mechanisms that help you maintain and regain equilibrium when upset or disturbed. In other words, your bodymind will seek out the state that allows for optimal functioning. Self-regulation is a natural and involuntary process that is controlled by the autonomic nervous system, which is the center of all unconscious functions within your bodymind.

**Self-regulation is the intelligence and power behind the
Welcoming-Process that frees what is blocked or stuck and naturally re-establishes *flow* and harmony within your bodymind.**

The innate self-regulating intelligence of your bodymind transforms and eventually harmonizes the contents of all of your experiences. Every time you welcome & allow your here and now experience the actual content begins to change and transform itself naturally and automatically. You don't need to *DO* anything other than be with what is. This work is designed to help you access the self-regulating intelligence within you that you may not have been shown how to access before.

**Self-regulation is the self-transforming and self-harmonizing
effect of the Welcoming-Process.**

With every additional Welcoming-Cycle the content of experience transforms even more and gradually begins to harmonize itself to the point that you feel at ease and more relaxed; especially when you compare your inner state with how you felt before you decided to approach the original issue or session theme.

The self-regulation mechanism of your bodymind causes the Actual-Allowing that, in turn, brings about the Bodyshift.

The Welcoming-Process is a not a loud, expressive practice. It is a very quiet, internal, and intimate procedure. In the moment of the actual-allowing when you notice the bodyshift, you automatically and naturally surrender to the self-harmonizing effect of the process.

The Bodyshift is the physical confirmation that the transformation has occurred in your bodymind.

THE WELCOMING-PROCESS IS
SELF-INTELLIGENT

Since the Welcoming-Process is a self-intelligent, self-transformative, and self-harmonizing process, you never know what will surface as you go through your Welcoming-Cycles. Although the process may seem simple, in practice it has an ingenious elegance that is very precise and specific to the needs of your bodymind.

Every time I use the Welcoming-Process I am surprised about the actual path the process takes. A wide array of experiential contents rises to the surface in ways I could never have predicted. The process has its own innate logic, however, and I eventually come to a plateau—a deep feeling of relaxation, peacefulness, and inner harmony. My experience has shown me that I always get to a deeper state of well-being. Sooner or later I always come to a place where I feel more loving towards myself, and more at peace with the session theme or issue. Sometimes I get there very quickly—after just two or three cycles—and sometimes it takes ten cycles or more. Each session is different and new. Your rational mind cannot figure out how a session will unfold and what the exact outcome will be. Given that the Welcoming-Process is self-intelligent and has a *mind of its own,* it cannot be figured out by rational thinking. All you need to do is start the process and keep repeating the Welcoming-Cycle until you reach a plateau; the transformation and harmonization of the session theme will automatically happen by itself.

"Anything you allow to be exactly as it is without trying to
change or fix it, will complete itself."
Ariel & Shya Kane

THE WELCOMING-PROCESS TRANSFORMS
YOUR SHADOW PATCHES

**The transformation of your shadow patches leads to an ever
greater realization of the presence of your inner sun—the source
of love & happiness within you.**

Consistent application of the Welcoming-Process will gradually transform and harmonize more and more of your shadow patches. As a result your
shadow layer *lightens-up* and becomes ever more transparent to the light of
your Inner Sun with its essential qualities.

The best way to recognize the self-harmonizing effect of the Welcoming-
Process is to pick an existing life challenge as your session theme. Then take
yourself through a complete written session. Once you reach the final plateau,
pause for a moment and compare your new state of being with your state at
the beginning of the session. When you feel a distinct difference in the quality
of your *overall state*, you are experiencing the self-harmonizing effect of the
Welcoming-Process. You can accentuate the benefits of this practice and reinforce your commitment to this path of Selflove by consciously taking note of
the positive changes.

As you read through the various Welcoming-Session examples in these
final chapters, it will become obvious that every person who applies the process
experiences these effects as a natural result.

DARREN DARES TO RELATE TO HIS EMOTIONAL BAGGAGE

This session was conducted over the phone. Before the session Darren said,
"I am so full of backed-up emotions that I'm afraid I'll explode or break down
if I don't get a release soon." I asked if he would like to be guided through an
entire Welcoming-Session. He accepted the offer and allowed me to guide him
through the process step-by-step. Here is a summary of what occurred:

Session Theme: "Exhaustion"

1. 1st Step - Welcoming: **"I feel hopelessness and resignation."**
   2nd Step - Allowing: Can you allow **this experience of hopelessness & resignation? No**
   Not-Allowing-Question: Can you allow **your No? Yes**
   3rd Step - Notice the Bodyshift as the Actual-Allowing occurs: **Deep exhalation**

2. 1st Step - Welcoming: **"Now, I feel anxiety."**
   2nd Step - Allowing: Can you allow **this anxiety? Yes**
   3rd Step - Notice the Bodyshift as the Actual-Allowing occurs: **Deep sigh**

3. 1st Step - Welcoming: **"I notice a sense of calmness & peace inside."**
   2nd Step - Allowing: Can you allow **this sense of calmness & peace inside of you? Yes**
   3rd Step - Notice the Bodyshift as the Actual-Allowing occurs: **Breathing is much slower**

1st Plateau:

After 3 minutes Darren reaches his first plateau. I ask him to orient. He says, "It's funny to be the observer of my eyes and to consciously notice how they roam around the room." As he orients, he keeps yawning. **"I feel very different. A real change has occurred, although we have only gone through three Welcoming-Cycles."** Then he decides to continue with the process because he feels there is more under this sense of peace.

4. 1st Step - Welcoming: **"I feel really tired & sleepy."**
   2nd Step - Allowing: Can you allow **feeling tired & sleepy? No**
   Not-Allowing-Question: Can you allow **your Not-Allowing? No (= 2nd No)***
   * Remember: if you answer also the Not-Allowing-Question with .... "No" then go back to the 1st Step of the Welcoming-Process and ask yourself the Welcoming-Question again.

5. 1st Step - Welcoming: **"My wanting to sleep is unacceptable to me."**
   2nd Step - Allowing: Can you allow **that your wanting is unacceptable?** <u>No</u>
   Not-Allowing-Question: Can you allow **your Resistance?** Yes
   3rd Step - Notice the Bodyshift as the Actual-Allowing occurs:
   My shoulders relax and sink down

6. 1st Step - Welcoming: **"I feel hungry."**
   2nd Step - Allowing: Can you allow **feeling hungry?** Yes
   3rd Step - Notice the Bodyshift as the Actual-Allowing occurs:
   A deep inhalation

7. 1st Step - Welcoming: **"I feel bored."**
   2nd Step - Allowing: Can you allow **feeling bored?** <u>No</u>
   Not-Allowing-Question: Can you allow **your No?** Yes
   3rd Step - Notice the Bodyshift as the Actual-Allowing occurs:
   Breathing deepens

8. 1st Step - Welcoming: **"My head and my body feel really separate."**
   2nd Step - Allowing: Can you allow **feeling this separation?** <u>No</u> Not-Allowing-Question: Can you allow **your Not-Allowing?** <u>No</u>
   (= 2nd No)*

9. 1st Step - Welcoming: **"My teeth are clenching and my forehead is throbbing."**
   2nd Step - Allowing: Can you allow **your clenching teeth and your throbbing forehead?** <u>No</u>
   Not-Allowing-Question: Can you allow **your Resistance?** <u>No</u>
   (= 2nd No)*

* If you say "No" to the Not-Allowing-Question (following the 2nd No-Rule) simply go back to the 1st Step of the Welcoming-Process and ask yoursel the Welcoming-Question.

10. 1ˢᵗ Step - Welcoming: **"I have an intense headache; my head is squashed in a vice."**
    2ⁿᵈ Step - Allowing: Can you allow **your head being squashed in a vice? Yes**
    3ʳᵈ Step - Notice the Bodyshift as the Actual-Allowing occurs:
    My head spontaneously tilts to the left and I take a deep breath

11. 1ˢᵗ Step - Welcoming: **"Now I feel really sad."**
    2ⁿᵈ Step - Allowing: Can you allow **feeling sad? Yes**
    3ʳᵈ Step - Notice the Bodyshift as the Actual-Allowing occurs:
    My cheeks sink lower and my bottom lip becomes heavier

12. 1ˢᵗ Step Welcoming: **"I get a weird looking image of a skull."**
    2ⁿᵈ Step: Allowing: Can you allow **this weird looking image? Yes**
    3ʳᵈ Step - Notice the Bodyshift as the Actual-Allowing occurs: **My body relaxes and I sink deeper into the mattress I am sitting on**

13. 1ˢᵗ Step - Welcoming: **"I am thinking about the movie I saw last night."**
    2ⁿᵈ Step - Allowing: Can you allow **this memory? Yes**
    3ʳᵈ Step - Notice the Bodyshift as the Actual-Allowing occurs:
    A sharp stinging sensation in my head

14. 1ˢᵗ Step - Welcoming: **"My head feels cloudy while I feel a ring of weight around it."**
    2ⁿᵈ Step - Allowing: Can you allow **this experience? Yes**
    3ʳᵈ Step - Notice the Bodyshift as the Actual-Allowing occurs:
    My body relaxes even more and I sink even more into the mattress

15. 1ˢᵗ Step - Welcoming: **"I feel at peace."**
    2ⁿᵈ Step - Allowing: Can you allow **this peace? Yes**
    3ʳᵈ Step - Notice the Bodyshift as the Actual-Allowing occurs: **Long deep and full breath**

16. 1ˢᵗ Step - Welcoming: **"I feel calmness and relaxation."**
2ⁿᵈ Step - Allowing: Can you allow this **experience? Yes**
3ʳᵈ Step - Notice the Bodyshift as the Actual-Allowing occurs: **Full breath**

2ⁿᵈ Plateau: While Darren is orienting himself by looking around in the room, he says: **"That was very cool. Compared to the beginning of the session I feel definitely better. I feel much calmer and my mind is very much in the present. My headache is also gone. I feel much more connected with this process. Now, I really know how it works from inside, based on my own experience."**

Session time: 30 minutes

THE PRINCIPLE OF NON-RESISTANCE

**"Nothing in the world is as soft and yielding as water,
yet nothing can better overcome the hard and strong,
for they can neither control nor do away with it."**
Lao Tse

The ancient Taoist Principle of *non-resistance* finds its fulfillment in the Welcoming-Process. Like water, the Welcoming-Process resists nothing; it only welcomes & allows your experience, just as it is. The welcoming & allowing steps are so open, so receptive, so inviting, so acquiescent, and so essentially loving in their nature that nothing can resist it. Because these simple steps, in effect, release any resistance you may have to your experiences, they are a practical application of this basic Taoist principle. Even your resistance, your aversion, your rejection—that inwardly felt *No!* that pushes against the content of your experience—is fully allowed by the 3 Not-Allowing-Questions. Resistance can only exist in a milieu of resistance. When there is nothing to push against, then resistance can no longer maintain its tense refusal. In the presence of this practical method, resistance can't help but naturally and automatically transform. This is what the Taoists have always understood and articulated as the principle of non-resistance.

Any resistance, any "no" that is welcomed & allowed automatically transforms and eventually harmonizes/ neutralizes itself based on the self-regulation effect of the Welcoming-Process.

Picture yourself pushing against another person's extended arm with all your force and weight. What do you sense in your body? Now, what happens if the other no longer resists, but gives in, by relaxing and dropping her/his arm? What happens with your resistance? Can you maintain it? No, because resistance can only maintain its resistance when there is something to resist against. The resistance automatically transforms and eventually neutralizes itself when it is fully received. The same is true with the content of your experience when it is fully welcomed & allowed.

The two following statements express the very same experiential fact:

"What you resist persists, what you experience disappears."
Werner Erhard

"What you resist, persists; what you accept, lightens."
Harold Bloomfield

As I mentioned in Chapter 3, we human beings have a tendency to reject and repress experiences we don't like, or that make us feel uncomfortable or scared. Unfortunately, what you resist or avoid goes underground and lives on in your shadow self, in the shadow layer of your bodymind. But what you consciously relate to, welcome and fully embrace, allow naturally and automatically transforms.

Eva Pierrakos conveys this principle quite beautifully in one of her *Pathwork Lectures:*

Through the Gateway

Through the gateway of feeling your weakness,
lies your strength.

Through the gateway of feeling your pain,
lies your pleasure and joy.

Through the gateway of feeling your fear,
lies your security and safety.

Through the gateway of feeling your loneliness,
lies your capacity to have fulfillment, love and companionship.

Through the gateway of feeling your hate,
lies your capacity to love.

Through the gateway of feeling your hopelessness,
lies your true and justified hope.

Through accepting the lacks of your childhood,
lies your fulfillment now.

Eva Pierrakos

The Welcoming-Process appeases the inner war by replacing self-rejection with receptivity in the Welcoming-Step and by replacing self-attack with the loving attitude of the Allowing-Step.

THE "LOVING FORMULA" OR THE "LOVING EQUATION"

What has been denied is being acknowledged.
What has been rejected is being invited.
What has been repressed is being welcomed.
What has been attacked is being embraced & allowed.
Welcoming & Allowing is a path of loving yourself and others,
and adopting a loving attitude toward all that is.

To Welcome & Allow = To Love

**To love yourself means that you welcome
& allow all of who you are, and all of your experiences,
including your resistance to their contents.**

How do you feel when somebody is fully present with you, *welcomes* you with full attention (Welcoming-Step), and then embraces all of you and what you share with an open heart (Allowing-Step), without trying to change you in any way? Take a moment and think of a person that you love. Now imagine this person would do just that for you: be totally present, giving you all of his or her attention and *completely allowing* you to be just as you are with all of your experiences regardless of their content? What do you feel when you imagine this?

This is my experience when somebody just welcomes & allows me as I am: "Wow, the other is really present, paying full attention, and completely receiving me as I am. I don't have to be any different. There is no need to protect myself. I can totally open up, say what I think and feel. I can just be as I am. I feel really understood, accepted, and cared for, actually loved."

On a physical level I notice how my breathing slows down and how I breathe ever more deeply from my belly. Simultaneously my muscles relax, my mind calms down, and I feel more present in my body as a sensation of ease and well-being begins to emerge. While I bask in the loving presence of the other I observe how a sense of peace and happiness wells up from within. In this moment life feels just wonderful.

Of course if you are emotionally upset or extremely agitated about something, it will take some time before you calm down, even in the presence of another. But if the other just keeps welcoming & allowing your experience as you share it, you will spontaneously move, more or less consciously, through various Welcoming-Cycles. Gradually your bodymind will calm down and you will reconnect with your inner center and the rays of the Inner Sun will begin to warm you from within.

Now that you know the *actual technique* of the Welcoming-Process, you can start to love yourself, by consciously welcoming & allowing all of your experiences, no matter how undesirable you find their content. Applying this process for yourself frees you ever more from the necessity of having to be loved by others. Of course it will still be wonderful and deeply fulfilling when someone loves you, but it is no longer a demand that you carry into every interaction. If you are being loved, that is great, and if not, that is okay, too. You still have your-self, and your own capacity to love yourself.

> **"The affirmation of one's own life, happiness, growth, and freedom is rooted in one's capacity to love."**
> Erich Fromm

THE "ACTUAL TECHNIQUE" OF THE WELCOMING-PROCESS

The *textbox-version* of the Welcoming-Process below is the linear description of the Welcoming-Cycle. I suggest that you make a copy of the Welcoming-Cycle on page 147, as well as the textbox-version, and use the one you like best until the whole process has become second nature to you.

---

1. **Welcoming: "What are you experiencing right now?"**
2. **Allowing: "Can you allow your here & now experience?"**

    1. If "Yes" go on to the 3rd Step of the Welcoming-Process
    2. If "No" ask one of the 3 Not-Allowing-Questions
    3. If your answer is "No" a second time (i.e., the 2nd No), re-start the Welcoming-Cycle & ask the Welcoming-Question again

3. **Noticing-the-Bodyshift – as the Actual-Allowing occurs**
4. **Keep repeating the Welcoming-Cycle until you reach a plateau**
5. **Write down your answer for each step!**

With the two copies handy you are ready to go ahead to the next chapter and practice the Welcoming-Process on your real life issues. But before you turn the page, acknowledge yourself for having come this far in learning the Art of Selflove!

CHAPTER 11

Now It's Your Turn!

"The key to understanding is always personal experience."
R.D.Laing

THE Welcoming-Process is exclusively experiential. It is much more than just a method or a technique. The Welcoming-Process is an *inner art*, a *way of life* that has its own intelligence, its own rhythm, and its own flow. But no matter how much you read about it or how much you try to understand it intellectually, you will only discover the deeper spirit when you begin to use it in the *laboratory* of your own bodymind.

Theories can help you to a point, but learning occurs through direct experience. There comes a moment when you have to jump, take that leap of faith and put what you have learned into practice. In other words, you will never truly know how to swim and what swimming feels like until you go into the water. The same is true for this process. Whatever my claims concerning its benefits may be, they won't mean much until they become a direct experience in your bodymind. I invite you now to jump, to get wet and immerse yourself in the *waters of your own experience* as you learn to swim through the challenges of daily life with the loving support of the Welcoming-Process.

"The soft overcomes the hard; the gentle overcomes the rigid. Everyone knows this is true, but few can put it into practice."
Lao Tse

Soon you will be *one of the few* who can put into practice what Lao Tse says by relating to your here and now experience with a conscious and loving attitude—the essence of practicing softness and gentleness in your own life.

The goal of this chapter is to give you all the remaining information in order to be fully equipped and capable of taking yourself through your first complete Welcoming-Session. After having read this chapter and completed your own session, you will be ready to start using the Welcoming-Process in all areas of your life, especially when you are confronted with challenging and emotionally upsetting situations.

The key to experiencing the real power of the Welcoming-Process is using it in daily life, particularly when your *buttons get pushed* and you feel emotionally triggered.

How to write down your own Welcoming-Sessions

"Writing down your Welcoming-Sessions consistently is the basis to mastering the Art of Selflove, as well as the guarantee that you will be capable of applying the Welcoming-Process spontaneously, *just in your head*, when you need it the most: in the middle of distressing situations of your daily life."

In this section you will be introduced to two versions of writing down your Welcoming-Session. Writing down each step is the most efficient way to ensure that Selflove becomes second nature, no matter where you are or what you are doing.

Two Basic Ways of Writing Down Your Welcoming-Session:

1. Regular Welcoming-Session Format
2. Short Welcoming-Session Format

The *Regular Welcoming-Session Format* will most likely be the only one you will use in the beginning until you have become thoroughly familiar with the process. After that you will only use the *Short Welcoming-Session Format*. Eventually you may create your own style and version of writing down your Welcoming-Sessions, which is a good thing to do.

1. Regular Welcoming-Session Format

Session Theme:

1. **1ˢᵗ Step - Welcoming:**
    2ⁿᵈ Step - Allowing: Can you allow...
    3ʳᵈ Step - Notice the Bodyshift as the Actual Allowing occurs:

You keep going by numbering each new Welcoming-Cycle (consisting of the 3 Steps of the Welcoming-Process) until you reach your 1ˢᵗ Plateau. Once you reach the plateau and have fully *oriented* yourself, decide if you want to go on or end your session at that point. If you carry on, keep numbering each Welcoming-Cycle until you reach the 2ⁿᵈ Plateau... and so on.

Example of a session excerpt using the Regular Format:

Session Theme: "Feeling lonely"

1. **1ˢᵗ Step - Welcoming:** "I feel a little lonely."
    2ⁿᵈ Step - Allowing: Can you allow feeling a little lonely? Yes
    3ʳᵈ Step - Notice the Bodyshift as the Actual-Allowing occurs: Deep inhalation

2. **1ˢᵗ Step - Welcoming:** "I long for tenderness and physical touch."
    2ⁿᵈ Step - Allowing: Can you allow this longing for tenderness and physical touch? No.
    2ⁿᵈ Step - Not-Allowing: Can you allow your Not-Allowing (No/ Resistance)? Yes
    3ʳᵈ Step - Notice the Bodyshift as the Actual-Allowing occurs: Yawning ...etc...

In the Appendix, on page 190, you will find a Regular Welcoming-Session Template that you can copy and use until you are ready to take yourself through a complete Welcoming-Session with the Short Welcoming-Session Format.

2. Short Welcoming-Session Format

W stands for **Welcoming-Step**
A stands for **Allowing-Step**
NBS stands for **Noticing-the-Bodyshift Step**

Example of a session excerpt using the Short Format:

Session Theme: "My Boss"

1) **W:** The fantasy comes up to go to the office of my boss and say in his face: "I have enough! I quit!"
   A: ...this fantasy/experience? Yes
   NBS: Deep breath & sigh, my whole body relaxes

2) **W:** "Tightness in my chest and closed down".
   A: ...this experience of tightness? No.
   Can you allow your No/Not-Allowing/Resistance? Yes
   NBS: Lengthening in the neck & relaxation in the shoulders... etc

Note: From here on all Welcoming-Sessions will be written up in the <u>Short Session Format</u>.

ARIELLE FACES HER SELF-CRITICISM

Arielle wrote down this session in her Selflove-Journal using the Short Session Format.

Session Theme: "Feeling stressed by my own criticism"

1) **W:** "I am angry at myself for not being more productive."
   A: experience? <u>No</u> **A:** <u>Not-Allowing?</u>* Yes **NBS:** Relaxation in my jaw
   * Can you allow your <u>Not-Allowing</u> of your experience?

2) **W**: "I feel sad." **A**: feeling of sadness? Yes **NBS**: Deep full breath

3) **W**: "I notice a deep calmness and stillness inside." **A**: experience? Yes **NBS**: Smiling & full breath

1ˢᵗ **Plateau**:

> Arielle's insight: **"It is easy to criticize myself when I feel afraid but much harder to relate to myself in a loving way."**

Session time: 5 minutes

RAVEN WELCOMES HIS EXISTENTIAL FEARS

What follows is a session I conducted over the phone with a client while he was recovering from a cancer operation and intense radiation treatments. He asked me to accompany him in his healing process by using the Welcoming-Process.

Session Theme: "Existential Fears"

These are Raven's words before we started the Welcoming-Session: **"I am afraid to lose all my money. I'm afraid to lose my health. I'm afraid of a recurrence of cancer. I am afraid of dying."**

1) **W**: "Tightness in my body and in my chest that makes me feel closed down." **A**: overall tightness? Yes **NBS**: Lengthening in the neck and relaxation in the shoulders

2) **W**: "I am feeling alone, separate & isolated." **A**: feeling alone, separate & isolated? Yes **NBS**: More space in my chest and in my head; especially behind my eyes

3) **W**: "Sadness and melancholy." **A**: experience? Yes **NBS**: Deeper breathing

Comments

Sometimes you might start a new Welcoming-Cycle while the bodyshift is still unfolding. The actual-allowing was quite profound and therefore ongoing in Raven's case. It is totally fine to start a new Welcoming-Cycle and make the still unraveling bodyshift the *next* content of experience you *welcome*, as Raven did in this session.

4) **W**: "I am feeling tingling and buzzing all over my body."
   A: sensations? Yes **NBS**: Yawning

5) **W**: "My whole body feels lighter… my skin is still buzzing."
   A: sensations? Yes **NBS**: Yawning several times in a row

6) **W**: "Energy has moved up from my legs to my pelvis and is even going to my neck"**A**: that energy has moved up in your body? Yes **NBS**: Deep breathing & more yawning

1ˢᵗ **Plateau**:

Raven: **"I feel more relaxed and there is more lightness in my head. I see a lighter color there. My original state definitely changed. Thoughts, emotions, and sensations have changed, and the physical tension has noticeably relaxed. I feel supported by the ground, and even by the mattress beneath me."** During his sharing Raven keeps yawning and stretching out his limbs.

Raven: **"I can observe even more bodyshifts occurring spontaneously, such as goose bumps and tingling. It feels like a *big plateau* to me. I no longer feel isolated. I feel more optimistic."**

Orienting during the plateau:

I invited Raven to consciously look around the room and out the window into the distance while closely observing *how the world looks* to him.

Raven: **"As I look around I notice a deeper breath coming up. I feel more grounded. All I want to do is just look around and to watch the sun come up. I just want to be."**

Check-in during the plateau:

After two minutes I asked Raven, "Raven, do you want to go on with the Welcoming-Session or do you feel it is enough for now?" He said, **"No! I feel ready to start my day! ...I am hungry."**

Session time: 20 minutes—including the sharing during the plateau.

> **"It is very helpful for me as a visual person to write down each step of the Welcoming-Process. I also like to put the "o.k. mark" once I can say, "Yes" to *allowing* my here and now experience."**
>
> Siegbert K. – a practitioner of the Welcoming-Process

Instead of writing Yes (Y) or No (N), you can just make a checkmark (√) for Yes, or a dash (–) for No

---

Now let's explore possible session themes that you could choose to work with using the Welcoming-Process.

THE BASIC 5 LIFE PILLARS:
CHOOSING A SESSION THEME

Each of the five pillars represents a major area of your life. The *5 Life Pillars* are:

- **Health and Body**
- **Work, Profession, and Creativity**
- **Relationships, Friendships, Family, and Social Life**
- **Money, Financial Security, and Material Comfort**
- **Meaning, Purpose, Personal Growth, and Spirituality**

Use the *5 Life Pillars* model to find a session theme any time you are not sure which issue you would like to work with. Simply remind yourself of the 5 Life Pillars and ask, "In which area of my life do I feel the most challenged or the least balanced?"

Or you might ask, "But what if I have no session theme?" It does not really matter if you have a session theme or not. You always start a Welcoming-Session right where you are, simply by asking, "What am I experiencing right now?"

The main difference between having and not having a session theme is the *entry point* that sets the *tone* of your session and gives it a basic direction. Most people like to pick a session theme because it enables them to track more easily the changes that occur, especially when they compare how they felt in the beginning versus at the end of the session in relation to the identified theme. At the same time, it is important to mention that even if you start out with a clear session theme, once you have asked the first Welcoming-Question you no longer have to focus specifically on the initial theme. So don't get bogged down with having or not having a session theme. What's important is to practice the Welcoming-Process and keep taking yourself through the various cycles until you reach a plateau.

Simply trust that the right contents of experience will naturally emerge, regardless of whether you start out with a session theme or not. Remember this process *works* because it makes use of the self-intelligent and self-regulating mechanisms of your bodymind.

When do you use the Welcoming-Process?

Whenever you feel challenged, emotionally upset, "triggered", or find yourself worrying about something, is the perfect moment to take out your Selflove-Journal and take yourself through a complete Welcoming-Session.

Every time you feel *off-balance*, disconnected from yourself, or emotionally stirred, this is an *internal call* of your bodymind to relate to yourself in conscious and loving way. Of course, you can apply it at any time, in any area of your life by choosing one of the 5 Life Pillars. But I have found that using this process when I feel emotionally *triggered* is by far the most powerful, most motivating, and most practical way of integrating the Art of Selflove into my daily life. I have come to realize that those moments when I am *not feeling at my best* is when I really need to give myself loving attention.

Once you have taken yourself through a complete session when you are feeling off-center, afraid, moody, upset, or whatever, the Welcoming-Process will no longer be something that you *should* do, but something you will really want to do. Your experience will show you how the self-harmonizing effect of this process almost magically transforms your initial disharmony and realigns you with your center. Using this process in this manner is no longer just another item on your to-do list, but truly a natural resource, like eating nourishing food, going for a walk out in nature, or taking a shower. Integrating the Welcoming-Process in this way will give you an ever greater sense of self-empowerment, ease, love, and happiness.

The emotional intensity scale

The *emotional intensity scale* is a simple method to evaluate the emotional intensity of your session theme or the current content of your experience. The scale ranges from 1 – 10, with 1 representing the lowest emotional intensity and 10 representing the highest level on the scale. When you are choosing a session theme, ask yourself, "On a scale from 1 – 10 how intense is my emotion about this theme?" The first intuitive response is the right answer. Below you are given an explicit explanation for each of the various intensity levels.

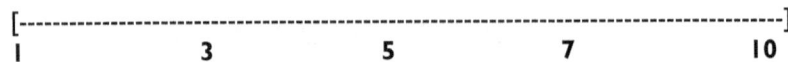

1-3: Quite neutral

The session theme, issue, or content of experience leaves you quite neutral. You can just observe and experience the session theme or the actual content of experience for what it is, in a neutral and almost emotionally detached way.

3-5: No longer neutral

The session theme, issue, or content of experience stirs up some emotions inside of you and you no longer feel neutral about it.

5-7: Emotionally triggered/feeling stressed

The session theme, issue, or content of experience triggers you emotionally and it absorbs a considerate amount of your energy and attention. You find yourself thinking about it often throughout the day and you are having many feelings about it that make you feel stressed inside.

7-9: Intensely triggered / feeling highly activated

The session theme, issue, or content of experience really *throws you off center*. You feel intensely triggered and highly activated. Emotionally you feel extremely stirred and your bodymind feels highly charged. It is hard to focus on anything else in the here and now because your mind is deeply absorbed in the issue. You *pull yourself together* because you are close to the edge of *emotionally bursting* or *acting out*.

10: Overwhelm—feeling powerless or helpless

The session theme, issue, or content of experience makes you feel completely *overwhelmed* or *powerless*. A 10 means that you can no longer handle the situation and that you are in need of professional help from a medical doctor, a psychiatrist, a psychologist, or any professional that knows how to deal with extreme states. Whenever you are faced with experiences that truly overwhelm you and surpass your current capacity to deal with them, then please, make sure you get professional support. Any time you feel trapped in a state that feels like a 10 it is of utmost importance to reach out and get professional help as soon as possible. If you have been exposed to a life threatening situation, you may go into a state of shock and feel *emotionally frozen* and internally paralyzed; this is an important time to seek professional help to work through the traumatic incident in a resourceful manner.

The Welcoming-Process is a practical method to cultivate a conscious and loving relationship with yourself; it is in no way a replacement for professional psychological or medical treatment.

IMPORTANT REMINDERS TO PREPARE FOR YOUR FIRST WELCOMING-SESSION

When you apply the Welcoming-Process for the first time you take a leap of faith. Each time you consciously welcome & allow your here and now experience you take a bit of a risk since you don't know what will happen in the process and what might come up as a result. As you keep going you might come to a similar realization as one client who said, "Wow, truly saying *Yes* to *allowing* my here and now experience, even if it feels uncomfortable in the beginning, does not really overwhelm me. On the contrary, as I keep going with the process, taking myself through further Welcoming-Cycles, the original session theme and its content of experience really transforms and eventually harmonizes itself."

And remember, you always have the option to use the built in safety valve of the Welcoming-Process by saying, *No* to *allowing* your here and now experience, especially when a certain content feels too intense, too uncomfortable, or too overwhelming to allow.

COPY & MAKE GOOD USE OF THE FRAMED TEXTBOXES & DIAGRAMS

I ask you now to either bookmark or make copies of the following textboxes and diagrams below—page numbers are indicated—and keep using them as support to take you by the hand and guide you through the Welcoming-Process until you know it by heart:

- **Summary of each of the 3 Steps of the Welcoming-Process** (p.106 / 124 & 135)

- **Diagram of the Welcoming-Cycle** (p.147)
- **"Actual Technique" of the Welcoming-Process given in a Textbox** (p. 164)
- **Regular or Short Welcoming-Session Format** (p. 169)
- **Regular Welcoming-Session Template** (p. 170)

Be gentle & patient with yourself

Remember to be patient with yourself as you learn to take yourself through complete Welcoming-Sessions, especially when you are dealing with challenging and stressful life situations. As with any new skill it takes some time to become proficient at it. In the beginning, when you learn skiing you will fall a lot and your style, the manner you come down the snowy slopes, will not look very elegant. Therefore give yourself the permission to take all the time you need to learn this new skill and be gentle with yourself in the process.

Let's Get Practical!

"What we have to learn to do, we learn by doing."
Aristotle

Now the moment has come to take yourself through your first complete Welcoming-Session. Use the written session format of your choice, either the Regular Welcoming-Session Format, on page 169 , or the Short Welcoming-Session Format, on page 170. The framed textbox below will give you the necessary instructions for successfully going through your first session.

How to do your first complete Welcoming-Session

1. **Get your Selflove-Journal and something you enjoy writing with.**

2. **Make sure you have <u>copies of these handy</u>:**

   - **Summary of each of the 3 Steps of the Welcoming-Process (p. 106 / 124 & 135)**
   - **Diagram of the Welcoming-Cycle (p.147)**
   - **The "Actual Technique" of the Welcoming-Process given in a Textbox (p.164)**
   - **Regular or Short Welcoming-Session Format (p.169 & 170)**

3. **Go to a place where you feel at ease and make yourself comfortable.**

4. **Take a few deep breaths into your belly; feel how your belly expands as you inhale and how it flattens as you exhale. Belly-breathing is calming and centers your awareness in your physical body.**

5. **Now, choose a session theme that challenges you, that you feel *uneasy* about or that *triggers* you emotionally.***

6. **Once you have chosen the session theme you are ready to start your Welcoming-Session. (Session format of your choice!) Begin with the first Welcoming-Cycle and keep going until you reach the 1st Plateau.**

   Have a good session!

* In the beginning, while you are still learning how to use the Welcoming-Process, only work with session themes on the emotional intensity scale of 3 – 5. When you have taken yourself through a few Welcoming-Sessions and are fairly familiar with the process, then you can begin to work with themes in the range of 5-7. Eventually when you feel really confident you can choose issues on the scale from 7-9.

GOOD LUCK WITH YOUR FIRST COMPLETE WELCOMING-SESSION!

Congratulations!

You have just completed your first entire Welcoming-Session!!!

Now you have all the necessary information and practical skills to cultivate the Art of Selflove. The more often you use the Welcoming-Process, the more you will deepen the experience of Selflove and happiness as the other benefits also begin to grace your day-to-day life.

**"Any genuine philosophy leads to action and from action back
again to wonder, to the enduring fact of mystery."**
Henry Miller

CHAPTER 12

Selflove -
Your Key & Path to a Fulfilling Life

The more loving you are with yourself, the happier you feel inside and the more loving you are with another, the happier they feel in your presence.

NOW, your Selflove journey really begins! Given that you are familiar with the Welcoming-Process and know how to love yourself and relate to your present experience in a conscious and loving way, you can freely use it in your daily life whenever you need it. The Welcoming-Process is a master key, a *passe-partout* that can open all the locks—even hidden doors and double-bolted gateways. Any obstacles you encounter on the path of Selflove can be surmounted with this process. The more you apply it the more doors will open up, the more your shadow patches and stress patterns will transform, and the more freely your Inner Sun will shine from within and radiate throughout your bodymind.

TAKING THE WELCOMING-PROCESS
TO THE NEXT LEVEL

This section shows you how you can get even more out the Welcoming-Process by taking it a step further still. Here is how you do it: several hours, days, or even weeks after you have completed a Welcoming-Session, take a moment to scan your written notes for statements, insights, creative ideas, or realizations that attract your interest or touch you emotionally. Mark these with a highlighter, or simply underline them with a colored pen so that they can easily be tracked as you browse through your Selflove-Journal. Then take some time and ponder these statements or insights. For example, you may have written something along these lines: "The thought of a new career makes me feel energized," or, "I feel angry when I don't express my needs in my partnership," or, "I miss spending more quality time with my family and loved ones." Generally, I recommend against reviewing your session in this manner right away. It is best to wait at least a few hours because you need space and time to integrate the changes that occur naturally after a session. As you contemplate the highlighted sentences you might gain even further insights or feel urged from within to make concrete changes in your life. Over the course of a few weeks or months, highlighting these key statements will help you see patterns and reveal those aspects in your life that truly demand your attention and require conscious action. Whatever the arena—be it career, relationship, health, or home—remember that the process is self-intelligent and brings into awareness whatever is imbalanced, neglected, overemphasized, or repressed. Some issues will naturally transform and harmonize while others will not get resolved, but keep coming up because they call for action in the outer world. The good news is this: if you keep looking for these key statements and insights in your sessions, this process will reveal previously unaddressed issues and recurring patterns.

If your outer life is really out of balance or in turmoil, then the agitation that results will trigger so much stress in your bodymind that the little-i will almost constantly respond in a reactive and fear-based manner. The first step toward reducing fear, worry, and distress is to begin to relate to yourself in a conscious and loving way. This is where the Welcoming-Process comes in. Go through the cycles and re-center yourself; then you can look at your situation from a calmer place. The appropriate next steps and practical decisions that will bring more stability and harmony to your external life will be easier to see when you are calm and centered. Sometimes this next step means reaching out to friends, family members, or professionals who can help you make the desired changes. Asking another person for support and to share her/his life experiences or professional expertise is an act of Selflove since you are making use of one of the most important resources in your life: other human beings.

At this point I would like to emphasize that the Welcoming-Process is not a religion, a philosophy, a moral codex, or set rules telling you how you *should* or *shouldn't* be and behave. In fact, it is quite the opposite because it allows you to tap into your inner authority and discernment. You are the master of your life and you decide how you want to live, what kind of changes you want to implement, and what sort of goals you want to achieve.

If we really love ourselves, everything in our life works.
Louise L. Hay

From a place of Selflove you are no longer motivated to be successful in order to gain admiration, status, or power but simply because realizing your goals is a natural expression and consequence of following the calling of your inner Self. As you continue loving yourself through various challenges, your self-confidence and self-esteem grows, as does your ability to pursue and realize your goals. By consciously integrating these newfound insights, discoveries, and intuitive hints gained in *reviewing* your Welcoming-Sessions you also prepare yourself to take the necessary steps to create more balance and fulfillment in your life.

SELFLOVE IS THE FOUNDATION TO CREATE LOVING RELATIONSHIPS WITH OTHERS

"If you love yourself, you love everybody else as you do yourself."
Master Eckhart

Have you ever asked yourself what the correlation is between loving yourself and loving another? The more loving you are with your*self*, the more loving you are with the *self* in others. Any content of experience that you love in yourself, you can also love in another. What you judge, hate, reject, and struggle with in yourself, you have a tendency to judge, hate, reject, and struggle with in another. What you have learned to understand and embrace in yourself, you can understand and embrace in others. If you are able to relate to your own anger, sadness, frustration, disappointment, and bad temper in a conscious and loving way, then you are better able to do the same with your fellow man or woman. The more you welcome & allow all of your experiences, including your resistance, the easier it is for you to welcome & allow the other person's experiences, too.

The way you love, hate, or fear yourself, is the way you love, hate, or fear another.

All of us long to be loved as we are. Nobody likes to be attacked, made wrong, or forced to change. What we really want in a relationship with another human being is to be *welcomed* and fully received—listened to, heard, felt, understood, and *allowed to be* exactly as we are. When you are present with a loving and conscious attitude for another person as she/he shares their experience they feel fully received and deeply understood, which automatically brings about relaxation and evokes an inner sense of lightness. In turn, the other person naturally feels *attracted* to you and begins to project positive feelings of ease and happiness onto you. Whether you are aware of it or not, the other cannot help but associate these *good feeling vibes* of love and happiness with you. Basically it is your *lovability*—your ability to love yourself and another human being—that makes you dear to others.

"The real bliss is how much you love yourself.
When you start to love yourself, you can love somebody else."
Sri Kaleshwar Swami

The cultivation of Selflove is a never-ending path, an ongoing process and continuous practice. You will never reach a final goal because there is always a deeper or higher level of *diving into the heart of your being-ness*. To love this deeply and fully is to unite the polar aspects that seem like opposites and become ever more whole. The more loving you are with yourself, the more you can experience harmony, happiness, and love inwardly, and the more you can share these qualities with others.

Truly loving yourself is truly loving another and truly loving another is truly loving yourself; because essentially there is only *One Self* – the Self in and out of which we all live.

The more you practice the Welcoming-Process, the more you will realize the One Self—the source of love and happiness—at the root or bottom of every experience, whatever its content.

THE WELCOMING-INVITATION OR AFFIRMATION

Remember, whenever you feel you have no choice but to attack yourself or get back at someone for what she/he did or didn't do, you know the little-i is running your life. Living from the *little-i* is a dead-end; you know this in your bones, and yet you may still fall into old patterns or feel driven to act out. The following affirmation is both an invitation and an effective reminder that will help you remember to use Welcoming-Process whenever you feel stressed, or catch yourself in the grip of a reactive behavior pattern.

"I feel *activated *right now,* so I simply *welcome & allow."*

---

* off-center, emotionally upset, distressed, moody, angry, frustrated, worried, anxious etc.

After saying the above statement, pause for a moment and take yourself through the Welcoming-Process until you reach a plateau; preferably in a written way with your Selflove-Journal. If circumstances don't permit you to write down your session, do the process in your head until you come back into balance and can interact from a centered state of being.

If you feel inspired to create your own *welcoming invitation or affirmation,* please feel free to do so.

FINAL WORDS

Congratulations, the Welcoming-Process is yours! Having gone through all the previous exercises you have acquired this lifetime skill. Now, you hold the key to inner happiness and loving relationships in your hand.

Please, be patient with yourself if you act out and behave in reactive ways occasionally. It takes a lot of practice to muster sufficient awareness, willpower, and intentionality to consciously observe and contain the highly charged survival energies in your bodymind. After years of practice, I still slip once in a while and catch myself in old habits like running away from uncomfortable situations or discharging reactive, blaming energy towards another rather than consciously relating to my current experience and taking full responsibility for it.

In contrast, every time I choose to welcome & allow an upsetting experience, I see the energy of its content transform and harmonize in my bodymind. On the other side of my resistance I find ease, relaxation and peace, and occasionally a blissful state of stillness. My ever renewing commitment to love myself—*no matter what*— is by far the most rewarding path I have ever embarked on. So, remember, there is no need for hurry or impatience, for every step towards Selflove is another step in the right direction towards greater freedom and harmony as more of your essential qualities shine forth.

Last but not least I would like to thank you for having traveled with me through the Art of Selflove. I feel grateful and honored to have had the privilege to share with you the Welcoming-Process. May it enrich you and everyone you relate with. I wish you a flourishing life full of love and happiness. Namaste—God bless you!

Appendix

"FINE-TUNING"

THIS appendix addresses common concerns about applying the Welcoming-Process in a Q&A format. Think of it as a fine-tuning manual. You can also look at the Q&A section on my website; I will regularly post answers to reader questions there. Also please feel free to e-mail me with any concerns that have not been answered in this book or on the website. Your questions, experiences, and feedback add to a growing body of knowledge gained from engaging with this process in real-time with real-life issues.

Is it okay to write up the Welcoming-Sessions in my own way—different from the regular or short session format ?

To write up your Welcoming-Sessions in your own style is not only okay, it is encouraged. Once we have mastered any basic skill, we tend to develop our own unique style. That's natural. The only thing I don't recommend is altering the actual process, because it may then lose its efficiency or not work at all. As long as you follow the basic steps and rules of the Welcoming-Process as outlined here, you will get good results. Writing down your sessions in your own way is a sure sign that this process is becoming second nature to you.

What do I do when I "feel stuck" during the Welcoming-Process?

If you feel stuck during the actual process, simply welcome the *feeling of "stuckness"* by making it the new content of your here and now experience. As you take yourself through a complete Welcoming-Cycle you will experience how the "stuckness" begins to transform and how you get back into the "flow" as you keep going with the process until you reach a plateau.

Example: "I feel stuck, nothing seems to move."

- **W:** "I feel stuck, nothing seems to move."
- **A:** ...feeling stuck and that nothing is moving? <u>No</u>.
- Can you allow your Not-Allowing/Resistance? Yes
- **NBS:** My whole body relaxes

What do I do when the same content of experience keeps coming up?

Sometimes a specific content of experience keeps resurfacing, for example: tiredness, moodiness, or worries in regard to an unresolved financial, relational, or health issue. That's natural and completely okay. Just continue welcoming & allowing this recurring content. With every additional Welcoming-Cycle, it will transform at an even deeper level, and eventually you will reach a plateau. Then, after you orient yourself, you can decide if you feel complete for the moment or if you want to continue your Welcoming-Session.

If the same session theme or content of experience keeps coming up over several days or weeks, then take your Selflove-Journal and do a review of your previous Welcoming-Sessions by marking crucial statements or insights in regard to the repeating pattern. Then reflect on these highlighted sentences and consider what concrete action steps are most appropriate for you to take in order to begin to resolve this issue in your life.

How do I deal with the "only-one-content rule" when a theme or experience suddenly emerges that is so important that I feel like writing down all of what is coming up?

The *only-one-content rule* is a guideline, and not set in stone. Sometimes you might be "on a roll." For example, you may have an intuitive insight, a creative idea, or be struck by a sudden revelation that moves you deeply. In this case it is totally okay and appropriate to write down all your thoughts and ideas before you go on to the 2nd Step of the Welcoming-Process. As long as you are not dealing with highly charged emotional issues, it is okay to make an exception to the only-one-content rule.

How many Welcoming-Cycles does it take to feel more at ease or to experience a substantial shift?

Sometimes it takes 15, 20, or even 30 Welcoming-Cycles before you experience a substantial change in your state of being. Depending on the emotional intensity or seriousness of the session theme or the content of experience you begin with, it will take more or less time or cycles before you notice a significant transformation and reach a plateau. At other times, just two or three cycles can create a substantial shift, even when dealing with a highly charged issue. The Welcoming-Session examples in this book will give you a good idea of how many cycles it generally takes to reach a plateau. And the reality is: you never know in advance how many cycles it will take, but if you keep going with the Welcoming-Process eventually you will experience the tangible harmonization and re-calibration that signals a plateau.

REGULAR WELCOMING-SESSION TEMPLATE

Session Theme: **Date:**

1) 1st Step - Welcoming:
   2nd Step - Allowing: Can you allow
   2nd Step - Not-Allowing: Can you allow your Not-Allowing/No/ Resistance?
   3rd Step - Notice the Bodyshift as the Actual-Allowing occurs:

2) 1st Step - Welcoming:
   2nd Step - Allowing: Can you allow
   2nd Step - Not-Allowing: Can you allow your Not-Allowing/No/ Resistance?
   3rd Step - Notice the Bodyshift as the Actual-Allowing occurs:

3) 1st Step - Welcoming:
   2nd Step - Allowing: Can you allow
   2nd Step - Not-Allowing: Can you allow your Not-Allowing/No/ Resistance?
   3rd Step - Notice the Bodyshift as the Actual-Allowing occurs:

4) 1st Step - Welcoming:
   2nd Step - Allowing: Can you allow
   2nd Step - Not-Allowing: Can you allow your Not-Allowing/No/ Resistance?
   3rd Step - Notice the Bodyshift as the Actual-Allowing occurs:

5) 1st Step - Welcoming:
   2nd Step - Allowing: Can you allow
   2nd Step - Not-Allowing: Can you allow your Not-Allowing/No/ Resistance?
   3rd Step - Notice the Bodyshift as the Actual-Allowing occurs:

_) 1st Step - Welcoming:
2nd Step - Allowing: Can you allow
2nd Step - Not-Allowing: Can you allow your Not-Allowing/No/ Resistance?
3rd Step - Notice the Bodyshift as the Actual-Allowing occurs:

_) 1st Step - Welcoming:
2nd Step - Allowing: Can you allow
2nd Step - Not-Allowing: Can you allow your Not-Allowing/No/ Resistance?
3rd Step - Notice the Bodyshift as the Actual-Allowing occurs:

_) 1st Step - Welcoming:
2nd Step - Allowing: Can you allow
2nd Step - Not-Allowing: Can you allow your Not-Allowing/No/ Resistance?
3rd Step - Notice the Bodyshift as the Actual-Allowing occurs:

_) 1st Step - Welcoming:
2nd Step - Allowing: Can you allow
2nd Step - Not-Allowing: Can you allow your Not-Allowing/No/ Resistance?
3rd Step - Notice the Bodyshift as the Actual-Allowing occurs:

_) 1st Step - Welcoming:
2nd Step - Allowing: Can you allow
2nd Step - Not-Allowing: Can you allow your Not-Allowing/No/ Resistance?
3rd Step - Notice the Bodyshift as the Actual-Allowing occurs:

_) 1st Step - Welcoming:
2nd Step - Allowing: Can you allow
2nd Step - Not-Allowing: Can you allow your Not-Allowing/No/ Resistance?
3rd Step - Notice the Bodyshift as the Actual-Allowing occurs:

Glossary

Actual-Allowing: This is the moment when the Bodyshift occurs. The Bodyshift itself comes about naturally and spontaneously. It cannot be willed, forced, or pushed in any way.

Allowing: This is the 2nd Step of the Welcoming-Process, consisting of the Allowing-Question: "Can you allow your experience?" & the Not-Allowing-Question: "Can you allow your No/Not-Allowing/Resistance?"

Attitude/Inner Attitude: This is your intentional or non-intentional *feeling-mind-set*, the inner stance or posture of how you relate to your here & now experience.

Big Eye: The symbolic representation of the inner observer that sees and notices all of your experiences in completely conscious, detached, and neutral mode.

Bodymind: A term that expresses the unity of the physical body and the mind/psyche, as well as the interplay between the physiological and psychological processes. Any change in the body will cause a change in the mind and vice versa. Bodymind is a common term that is used by authors such as Ken Dychtwald in *Bodymind* and Ethan Miller in *Bodymind.*

Body-Sensation: The physical phenomenon that you feel in your body. I've included a list of the different types of body-sensations on page 60. Becoming aware of your body-sensations is also the foundation to *Notice the Bodyshift*, the 3rd Step of the Welcoming-Process.

Bodyshift: This is the body signal—the involuntary, physical change, (i.e. a sudden, unexpected inhalation or exhalation, yawning, or giggling) which occurs in your body in the moment of the Actual Allowing. The Bodyshift is the feedback step of the Welcoming-Process, the confirmation that the Actual Allowing has occurred, that your Bodymind has fully allowed the content of your experience.

Flower of Experience: An illustration that shows all the 5 Elements of Experience in the shape of a flower with the center position occupied by the Inner Observer.

Inner Critic: The voice in your head that judges you based on some idealized notion of good/bad, right/wrong, should/shouldn't. This negative self-talk shames and condemns you and this, in turn, undermines your sense of self and therefore your sense of self-esteem, self-worth, and self-confidence.

Inner Observer: The awareness within you, the conscious "I" that simply watches *what is* from a neutral, witness stance. It is the part of your conscious personality that is not identified with any of your experiences.

little-i: The part in you that is fully identified with the content of your experience and believes that what you experience defines who you are. Being completely absorbed in the content of your experience it responds in a reactive and habitual manner. See the diagram, *The Reactive Behavior Pattern of the little-i* on page 82.

Loving Equation/Loving Formula: To Welcome & Allow = To Love (Expressed in words, "To love" means "to welcome & allow".)

Noticing-the-Bodyshift: This is the 3rd Step of the Welcoming-Process. You bring your awareness into your body and observe your body-sensations until you notice the change that occurs in the moment of the Actual Allowing.

Orienting: Consciously looking at the shapes, colors, and structures of the objects in your environment you are instinctively drawn to while you are fully enjoying your plateau. *Orienting* automatically invites your nervous system to *bridge* the perception of your inner and outer world and thus creates a natural balance between the two.

Plateau: The *resting phase* that you automatically come to in a Welcoming-Session after having completed a certain number of Welcoming-Cycles. The Plateau is also an *integration phase* that provides you with the opportunity to absorb and incorporate the *harmonizing after-effects* of the Welcoming-Process.

Plateau-Rule: means that in order to do a complete Welcoming-Session you go through as many Welcoming-Cycles until you reach a relaxed or balanced state of being—a stable, internal resting place.

Sensory-Perception: An impression coming from the external world registers through sight, smell, touch, taste, or hearing.

Selflove: The natural unity of Love and Self on the essential level of your being, the very existence of who you are; your true SELF. It is also the radiant essence streaming out of you, as well as the process of loving yourself as a resource and a foundation upon which to live and grow.

Self-Regulation: An *intelligent process* inherent in your Bodymind that automatically transforms & harmonizes any content of your experience that you welcome & allow. Similar to the way your physical body regulates itself by maintaining *homeostasis*, your psyche has its own way of maintaining balance and equilibrium by adjusting and recalibrating as needed.

Soma: A Greek term that means, "the body experienced from within." Soma and Bodymind are interchangeable terms as both indicate that body and mind form a functional unit and are not wholly separate by nature.

Session Theme: This is the issue that you choose to work with in your Welcoming-Session.

Welcoming: This is the 1st Step of the Welcoming-Process, consisting of the Welcoming-Question: What are you experiencing right now?

Welcoming-Cycle: The *heart* and summary of the central technique herein discussed, as well as a simplified illustration and summary of how the 3 steps work together in a circular system.

5 Elements of Experience:

1. Body-Sensations & Sensory-Perceptions
2. Needs & Desires
3. Emotions & Feelings
4. Thoughts, Ideas, & Concepts
5. Images, Fantasies, Memories, Stories, & Dreams

References

Chapter 1

1. Babaji Nagaraj, "Weekly Message #182: Babaji's Kriya Yoga," ed. Sonia Giguère. http://www.babajiskriyayoga.net
2. Swami Prajnanpad, "Die Weisheit Indiens" Trans. into German by Danielle & Olivier Föllmi (März, ISBN 3-89660-234-9) Knesebeck Verlag Presse, 2003

Chapter 2

1. Ernest Holmes, "The Science of Mind," 478. Tarcher/Putnam, 1998
2. Paramahansa Yogananda, "The Divine Romance," Back Cover. Self-Realization Fellowship, 2000
3. Aristotle, "Quote on Happiness," http://www.cybernation.com
4. Asian Saying, freely quoted from memory
5. Dionne Marx, Foreword to *The Philosophy of Love*, by Haridas Chaudhuri, xiv. Routledge & Kegan Paul, 1987
6. Excerpt from the Tablets of Shambala, http://www.mahendranath.org/levogyrate.mhtml.
7. Theilard de Chardin, Quote from "Exploring Meditation," Dr. Susan G.
   Shumsky, 231. The Career Press. Inc., 2002
8. Siva Yogaswami of the Natha Sampradaya,
   Quote: http://www.angelfire.com/hi/HSCatYORK/a5.html
9. Lester Levenson, "Keys to the Ultimate Freedom," 50. Sedona Institute, Phoenix, Ariz., 1993
10. Daniel Odier, "Desire", 231. Inner Traditions, 2001

11. Dionne Marx, Foreword to *The Philosophy of Love*, by Haridas Chaudhuri, ix Routledge & Kegan Paul, 1987
12. Translation of Saccidananda or Sat-cit-ananda, Wikipedia Encyclopedia. http://en.wikipedia.org/wiki/Satchitananda
13. Maharishi Mahesh Yogi, "Bhagavad Gita – A New Translation and Commentary," 100 & 102. Arakana, 1990
14. Carl Gustav Jung, "The Collected Works of C.G. Jung," CW 12, par. 44. Routledge and Kegan Paul, 1953
15. Carl Gustav Jung, "The Collected Works of C.G. Jung," CW 7, par. 404. Routledge and Kegan Paul, Ltd, 1953
16. Marshall Govindan & Jan Ahlund, "Kriya Yoga: Insights Along the Path," 107. Babaji's Kriya Yoga & Publications, Inc, 2008

CHAPTER 3

1. Francis Meehan, Quote: http://www.cybernation.com
2. David Boadella & David Smith, "Maps of Character", 56. Abbotsbury Publications/England
3. Nathaniel Branden, "Honoring the Self," 172. Bantam Books, 1985
4. Susan Thesenga, "The Undefended Self," 68. Self Published, 1988
5. Carl Gustav Jung, "Man and His Symbols," 83. Dell Publishing, 1968
6. Carl Gustav Jung, "The Collected Works of C.G. Jung," CW 9i, par. 513. Routledge and Kegan Paul, 1953
7. Carl Gustav Jung, "The Collected Works of C.G. Jung," CW 9ii, par. 422. Routledge and Kegan Paul, 1953
8. Tenzin Wangyal Rinpoche, "The Tibetan Yogas of Dream and Sleep," 29. Snow Lion Publications, 1993
9. V.T. Neelakantan, S.A.A. Ramaiah, Babaji Nagaraj, "The Voice of Babaji,", 115. Babaji's Kriya Yoga Order of Acharyas, Inc., 2003
10. Hal & Sidra Stone, "Embracing Your Inner Critic," 9. Harper San Francisco, 1993
11. Nathaniel Branden, "Honoring the Self," xi. Bantam Books, 1985
12. Oprah Winfrey, Quote: http://www.cybernation.com
13. A Course In Miracles, Quote: http://www.cybernation.com

14. Eva Broch-Pierrakos-Pathwork, "Lecture # 83 – April 14, 1961, earlier printed version," p. 4
15. African Proverb, Quoted by Les Brown in his speech, "Live Full – Die Empty," http://www.SeminarsonDVD.com

CHAPTER 4

1. Italian Proverb, Quote: http://www.cybernation.com
2. Lao Tse, Quote: http://thinkexist.com/quotation/knowing_others_is_wisdom-knowing_yourself_is/148363.html
3. Marshall Govindan, "The Yoga Sutras of Patanjali and the Siddhas," 206-207. Kriya Yoga Publications, 2001
4. Abraham Maslow, Citation: http://en.wikipedia.org/wiki/Abraham_Maslow
5. Robert Plutchik, http://www.personalityresearch.org/basicemotions/plutchik.html and http://en.wikipedia.org/wiki/Robert_Plutchik
6. Marshall Govindan & Jan Ahlund, "Kriya Yoga: Insights Along the Path," 29. Babaji's Kriya Yoga & Publications, Inc., 2008
7. Panayota Theotoki-Atteshli, "Gates to the Light," 13. Printed by IMPRINTA Ltd., 1996
8. Lester Levenson, Opening Quote to "Keys to the Ultimate Freedom," Sedona Institute, Phoenix, Ariz., 1993

CHAPTER 5

1. William James, Quote: http://*www.quoteworld.org/quotes/7113*
2. William Shakespeare, Quote: www.brainyquote.com/quotes/quotes/w/williamsha109527.html
3. Peter Levine, "Waking the Tiger/Healing Trauma," 87-88. North Atlantic Books Berkeley, California, 1997
4. Epictetus, Quote: http://www.cybernation.com
5. W. Clement Stone, Quote: http://www.cybernation.com
6. Viktor E. Frankl, Quote: http://www.cybernation.com
7. Quote from Unknown Source: http://www.cybernation.com
8. Charlotte Selver, "Pioneering teacher of Sensory Awareness," Quote http://www.cybernation.com

9. Charles Swindoll, Quote: http://www.cybernation.com
10. Tom Blandi, Quote: http://www.cybernation.com

CHAPTER 6

1. APA (American Psychology Association), "Open Up! Writing About Trauma Reduces Stress, Aids Immunity," Psychology Matters. www.psychologymatters.org/pennebaker.html, (accessed March 23, 2009)

CHAPTER 7

1. John 8:31-32, New International Version.
2. Aesop (620-560 BC), Quote: http://www.cybernation.com
3. Lao Tse, Quote (restated in the present): http://www.theotherpages.org/quote/alpha-t4.html
4. Tara Bennet-Goleman, "Emotional Alchemy," 169. Harmony Books, 2001

CHAPTER 8

1. Rumi, Quote from "Boundless Happiness," Miranda Holden, 162. Rider Books, 2002
2. Henry Miller, Quote: http://www.cybernation.com
3. Nathaniel Branden, Quote: http://www.cybernation.com
4. Ariel & Shya Kane, "Magical Relationship," 30. Ask Productions, Inc., 2006
5. Will Garcia, Quote: http://www.cybernation.com
6. Werner Erhard, Quote: http://www.cybernation.com
7. Denis De Rougemont, Quote: http://www.cybernation.com

CHAPTER 9

1. Excerpts from, "The incredible, communicable yawn," http://www.seedmagazine.com/content/article/the_incredible_communicable_yawn/ (accessed July 12, 2009)

Chapter 10

1. Black Elk, Oglala Sioux, "Native American Wisdom" Running Press, 1994
2. Carl Gustav Jung, "Analytical Psychology—It's Theory and Practice," Vintage Books, 1995
3. Ariel & Shya Kane, "Magical Relationship," 28. Ask Productions, Inc., 2006
4. Lao Tse, "Translation of the Tao Te Ching," translated by Peter Merel, excerpt from the 78th stanza, http://www.religiousworlds.com/taoism/ttcmerel.html
5. Werner Erhard, Quote from, "Characterological Transformation," Stephen M. Johnson, 229. W.W. Norton, New York/London, 1985
6. Harold Bloomfield, "Love Secrets for a Lasting Relationship," 82. Bantam Books, 1994
7. Eva Broch-Pierrakos, "Guide Lecture #190," http://www.pathwork.org/lectures/P190.pdf
8. Erich Fromm, "The Art of Loving," 50. Perennial Library, Harper & Row, 1962

Chapter 11

1. R.D. Laing, Quote from VHS, "Eros, Love, & Lies," Release: 1990 – USA
2. Lao Tse, "Translation of the Tao Te Ching," translated by Stephen Mitchel, excerpt from the 78th stanza, http://www.terebess.hu/english/tao/mitchell.html#Kap78
3. Aristotle, Quote: http://www.cybernation.com
4. Henry Miller, Quote: http://www.cybernation.com

Chapter 12

1. Louise L. Hay, Quote: http://www.cybernation.com
2. Meister Eckhart, translated by R.B.Blakney, 204. Harper & Brothers, 1941
3. Sri Kaleshwar Swami, excerpt taken from his webpage: http://www.kaleshwar.org/en/store_book_dattakriya

Acknowledgement

would like to thank my mother, Marie-Louise, for teaching me that *love* is the central principle of life, my father, Dieter, who died before I was able to speak with him, my ancestors for their legacy, especially my grandparents, who have been the inspiration, guidance, and sweetness in my early years, Daniela Koenig for her loving support and her editing input, Caitlin Catley for believing in me and my book project, my brother, Adrian, who keeps me grounded by confronting me with the "hard facts" of life, Valérie for advising me to start writing in English, and Tekeal Riley, my first conscious relationship teacher. And a special thank you to my *professional book-team*: Sandra England for her feedback on my first manuscript, Geralyn Gendreau, my editor, for her creative input and professional support in my writing process, Sam Roberts for designing the entire book cover and giving my diagrams a professional look, Robine Yohm for her meticulous proofreading job, Robin Meyers for the back cover copywriting, Art Durand for my back cover picture, and Bob Powers, Jonathan Gullery and their colleagues at R.J. Communications for printing and distributing my book.

Furthermore I feel grateful for all my friends, family members, and personal teachers in body and spirit who have enriched my life: Raven Jones, Max J. van Praag, Gabriela Fritschi, Jürg Ott, Bernhard Maul, Mukul Kumar, Roger K. Marsh, Alice & Louise Lobsiger, Patricia Elwood, Andrea-Katja Lobsiger, Liliana Acero, Carol Spirig, Martin & Judith Mueller, Walter Orion, Darren Stamos, Silvana Pagani, Rosemary Shoong, Wil Bullock, Michael Flemming, Rolf Steiner, Annicka Hentonnen, Lukas Wiesli, Corinne Zobrist, Anne-Françoise Cart, Amr Huber, Karri Karrer, Maggi Gonzalez, Reinhold Knips, Norbert Soentgen, Siegbert Kiessler, Norbert Geiger, Whitney Gordon, Noi, Kalsang Choedon, the New York Pathwork community, the Biosynthesis T9 members, David Boadella, Silvia Specht-Boadella, Peter Levine, Steve Hoskinson, Barbara Brennan, Eleanor Criswell-Hanna, Lee Glickstein, Marshall Govindan Satchidananda, Nandhi, Kriyananda, Sri Siva,

Sri Kaleshwar, Sanaya Roman, Duane Packer, Paramahansa Yogananda, Babaji Nagaraj, Baird T. Spalding, C.G. Jung, Lester Levenson, Jane Roberts, and everyone who has enriched my life that I did not mention by name.

My deepest gratitude goes to all the Beings of Light, the Siddhas—the perfected yogi-masters—and the Divine—The-All-That-Is—the innermost Self, in and out of which we all live and that keeps nurturing, guiding, and blessing our lives and all of existence in the eternal now.

Thank You All!

CONTACT INFORMATION

For Individual Phone-/Skype-Coaching Sessions, Online-Seminars & Live SelfLove-Trainings go to:

www.TheArtofSelfLove.com

E-mail: FrankLobsiger@TheArtofSelfLove.com
Phone (CH): ++41 (0) 26 670 3324

www.ingramcontent.com/pod-product-compliance
Lightning Source LLC
Chambersburg PA
CBHW071733120626
46550CB00002B/506